Hoberman/May

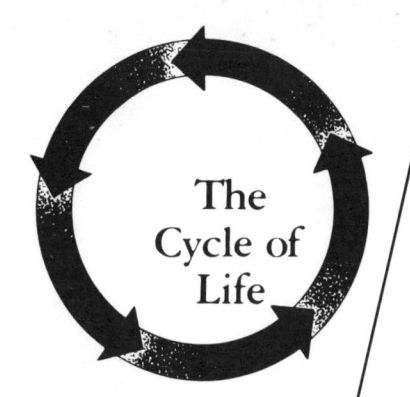

The Cycle of Life

Guide to
PARENTING:
You and Your
NEWBORN

ALSO BY DONNA HOHMANN EWY AND RODGER FRANK EWY:

Preparation for Childbirth

Preparation for Breastfeeding

The Cycle of Life
Guide to a Healthy Pregnancy
Guide to Family-centered Childbirth

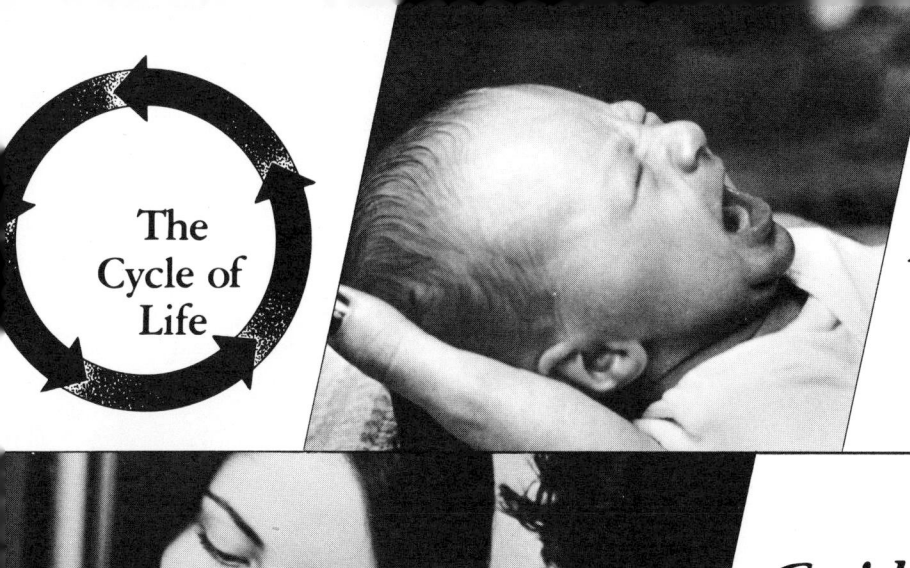

The Cycle of Life

Donna and Rodger Ewy

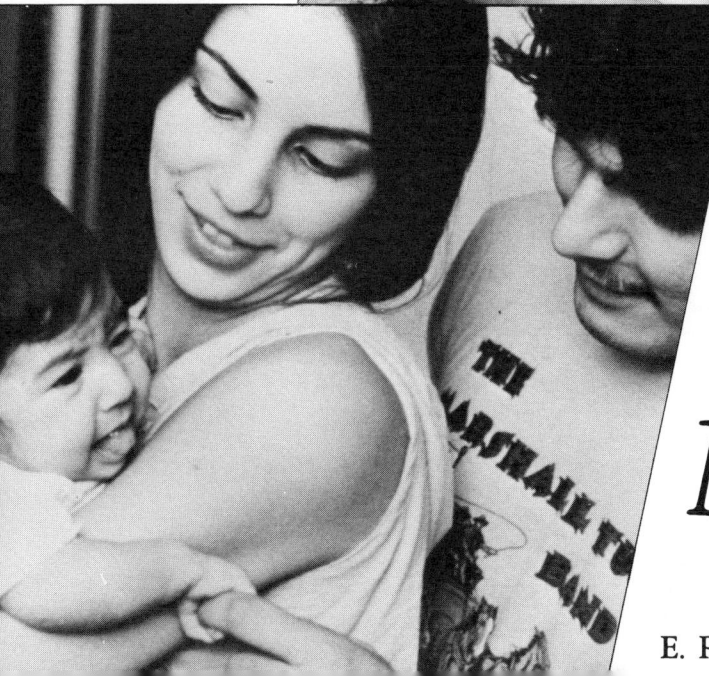

Guide to
PARENTING:
You and Your NEWBORN

E. P. DUTTON / NEW YORK

Copyright © 1981 by Donna and Rodger Ewy / All rights reserved. Printed in the U.S.A. / No part of this publication may be reproduced or transmitted in any form or by any means, electronic or mechanical, including photocopy, recording or any information storage and retrieval system now known or to be invented, without permission in writing from the publisher, except by a reviewer who wishes to quote brief passages in connection with a review written for inclusion in a magazine, newspaper or broadcast / Published in the United States by E. P. Dutton, Inc., 2 Park Avenue, New York, N.Y. 10016 / Library of Congress Cataloging in Publication Data / Ewy, Donna / Guide to parenting / (The Cycle of life; v. 3) / Bibliography: p. 143 / Includes index. / 1. Parenting—United States. 2. Infants—Care and hygiene—United States. 3. Infant psychology—United States. I. Ewy, Rodger. II. Title. III. Series: Ewy, Donna. Cycle of life; v. 3 / HQ755.8.E973 1981 / 649'.122 / 81-9842 / ISBN: 0-525-93184-8 / AACR2 / Published simultaneously in Canada by Clarke, Irwin & Company Limited, Toronto and Vancouver / 10 9 8 7 6 5 4 3 2 1 / First Edition

To Donna's father

Lee Hohmann

who loved children

and passed on a special heritage of love

to his children and grandchildren

so that future generations may inherit

the precious gift he left with us

Newborn's Ten Commandments to Parents

Dear Parent:

I come to you a small, immature being with my own style and personality. I am yours for only a short time; enjoy me.

1. Please take time to find out who I am, how I differ from you and how much I can bring to you.
2. Please feed me when I am hungry. I never knew hunger in your uterus, and clocks and time mean little to me.
3. Please hold, cuddle, kiss, touch, stroke, and croon to me. I was always held closely in your uterus and was never alone before.
4. Please don't be disappointed when I am not the perfect baby that you expected, nor disappointed with yourselves that you are not the perfect parents.
5. Please don't expect too much from me as your newborn baby, or too much from yourselves as parents. Give us both six weeks as a birthday present—six weeks for me to grow, develop, mature and become more stable and predictable; and six weeks for you to rest and relax and allow your body to get back to normal.
6. Please forgive me if I cry a lot. Bear with me and in a short time, as I mature, I will spend less and less time crying—and more time socializing.
7. Please watch me carefully and I can tell you those things which soothe, console

and please me. I am not a tyrant who was sent to make your life miserable, but the only way I can tell you that I am not happy is with my cry.
8. Please remember that I am resilient and can withstand the many natural mistakes you will make with me. As long as you make them with love, you cannot ruin me.
9. Please take care of yourself and eat a balanced diet, rest and exercise so that when we are together you have the health and strength to take care of me.
10. Please take care of your relationship with each other, for what good is family bonding if there is no family to bond to?

Although I may have turned your life upside down, please realize that things will be back to normal before long.

Thank you,
Your loving child

Contents

    Acknowledgments   *x*
    Introduction   *xii*
1. The Importance of the Family   *1*
2. What Kind of Parent Will You Be?   *5*
3. Your Newborn   *13*
4. Soothing Your Newborn   *33*
5. Playing with Your Newborn   *41*
6. Feeding Your Newborn   *47*
7. Caring for Your Newborn   *61*
8. Common Concerns of New Parents   *73*
9. Mother's Recovery After Delivery   *81*
10. At Home—Daily Care and Nutrition   *93*
11. Postnatal Exercises   *107*
12. Changing Roles   *115*
13. Your Marriage   *127*
    Glossary   *137*
    Further Reading   *143*

Acknowledgments

We would like especially to thank the following people who shared their time, energy, and information with us:

First, our parents who gave us our first important lessons in parenting. Next, our children Marguerite, Suzanne, Rodger, and Leon, who have unceasingly tested our own parenting techniques and given us invaluable experiences.

Our special appreciation goes to the many pregnant parents who have shared their experiences and families with us: Ann and Sam Baron, Anne and K. L. Berry, Minnie Cordova, Anita and Andre DePriest, Lynn and Ken Ewall, Tommy and Ron Farina, Gail and Dave Hall, Kathy and Mike Hinojos, Mike and Cecile Lederhos, Ted and Stacey Levin, Linda Loeb, Sherry Mulloy, Jeannie Paxton, Jim and Donnette Raabe, Roberta and Bob Scaer, Robyn and Rick Sears, Peggy Smith, Dennis Surina, Kay Wilson, and Cindy Yeoman.

We are especially grateful for the information and critiques shared so generously by our professional consultants: Kathy Bernau, R.N., M.S., Coordinator of Patient Education, Rose Medical Center, Denver; Watson Bowes, Jr., M.D., Chairman, Department of Obstetrics / Gynecology, University of Colorado School of Medicine, Denver; T. Berry Brazelton, M.D., Chief, Child Development Unit, The Children's Hospital Medical Center, and Associate Professor of Pediatrics, Harvard Medical School, Cambridge; Joseph Butterfield, M.D., Chairman, Department of Perinatology, Children's Hospital, Denver; William Clewell, M.D., Assistant Professor of Obstetrics / Gynecology, University of Colorado School of Medicine, Denver; Harvey M. Cohen, M.D., Department of Obstetrics / Gynecology St. Anthony's Hospital, Denver; Robert Emde, M.D., Professor of Psychiatry, University of Colorado School of Medicine, Denver; Bob Harmon, M.D., Assistant Professor of Child Psychiatry, University of Colorado School of Medicine, Denver; Trudy Hutchinson, Registered Dietician, Nutrition Service, University of Colorado Medical Center, Denver; Betty Jennings, Certified Nurse Midwife/Practitioner, Obstetrics Clinic, University of Colorado Medical Center, Denver; William Kimberling, Ph.D., Assistant Professor of Genetics, Department of Pediatrics, University of Colorado School of Medicine, Denver; Marshall H. Klaus, M.D., Professor of Pediatrics, Case Western Reserve University, Cleveland; Mary Krugman, R.N., M.S., Coordinator of Parent Education, Rose Medical Center, Denver; Richard Krugman, M.D., Associate Professor of Pediatrics, Codirector of Child Health Associate Program, University of Colorado School of Medicine, Denver; Heidi Lynch, R.P.T., C.C.E., American Society for Psychoprophylaxis in Obstetrics Trainer, Boulder; Patricia O'Connor, R.N., C.C.E., Assistant Coordinator, Nurses Association of the American College of Obstetricians and Gynecologists, Vice Chairman, American Society for Psychoprophylaxis in Childbirth, Denver; Doug Pugh, M.D., Clinical Neonatology Fellow, Division of Perinatal Medicine, University of Colorado Medical Center, Denver; Reva Rubin, Professor, Department of Maternity Nursing, University of Pittsburgh; Pamela Shrock, R.P.T., M.P.M., Clinical Nurse Consultant, Chicago; Vicki Walton, Manager, The Birthplace, Seattle; Paul Wexler, M.D., Chairman, Dept. of Obstetrics / Gynecology, Rose Medical Center, Denver and Assistant Clinical Professor, University of Colorado School of Medicine, Denver; and Marelynn W. Zipser, Ph.D., Nutritionist.

Paula Lehr and Rebecca Metcalfe have our great appreciation for the many hours they spent at the typewriter.

To our editors, Sally Crowley, Patti Hodgins, Marian Skedgell, Karen Braziller, and Amelie Littell, our thanks for their important contributions.

Finally, we would like to thank our good friend Warren Rovetch, who had the vision to see in print the books *Cycle of Life: Guide to a Healthy Pregnancy, Guide to Family-centered Childbirth,* and *Guide to Parenting: You and Your Newborn.*

Introduction

Guide to Parenting: You and Your Newborn was developed to fill the information gap about newborns from the moment of birth through the difficult first six weeks.

Your baby's temperament and personality influence your style of loving and coping. This in turn affects your infant. It is a constant cycle that starts in the very first days. From the moment of birth, your baby has the ability to send messages to indicate her needs and to initiate social activity with you. These social interactions are as important to your baby as food and sleep. Infants who can send out clear cues make parenting an enjoyable task. Those infants who have difficulty communicating their needs are more of a challenge to their parents.

As a mother of a newborn, your emotions may range from great joy to feelings of despair. You are especially vulnerable at this time. Your self-esteem and how you feel about yourself in the mothering role are vital to your love and attachment to your baby. Your baby's behavior and responses to your efforts influence you from the first hours of her life. If your baby is responsive, cuddly, soothable and predictable, you will feel good about your mothering role. If your baby is nonresponsive, inconsolable, and erratic, you may feel concerned about your ability to mother and must develop extra sensitivity to your baby's needs to help her respond to your efforts.

You, the father, are also greatly affected by your baby's personality and behavior. An alert baby influences how you feel about yourself and your wife. A responsive baby helps you feel you are a good father and your wife is a successful mother.

Fulfilling your baby's physical needs is only one part of parenting. Being there to soothe and stimulate her when she needs you and being able to communicate your love and receive her love is the essence of parenting with joy.

Mothering and fathering are your most crucial tasks as new parents. Like every mother and father, you want to be successful parents and enjoy your newborn. Success does not rest with you alone, however. You and your child interact constantly. In early parenting, your baby shapes your behavior by her responses to your efforts. Only toward the end of the first year do you, the parent, begin to shape your baby's behavior.

Recently, there has been a great deal of research on how newborns and their parents relate to each other. Dr. T. Berry Brazelton has shown us that not only can the newborn see, but prefers and can follow the human face at birth. Klaus described the significance of the first hours and days of life. Wolff explored the significance of the states of consciousness in a newborn. Reva Rubin explored the importance of the maternal tasks a mother undergoes during pregnancy and birth. Lang showed that a newborn can hear and turns to and follows a human voice, preferring a high-pitched voice at birth. Condon and Sander demonstrated the synchronization between mother and baby, and described how a baby tunes into and moves in rhythm with human speech. Sanders explained that a steady routine in early days helps the newborn to adapt to life outside the uterus. MacFarlane illustrated the ability of an infant to discriminate the odor of the mother's breast pad by the fifth day. Philips discovered that a baby placed at the mother's breast, with skin-to-skin contact, shows a minimal drop in body temperature. Metzoff and Moore demonstrated that newborns can imitate tongue and lip movements, open their mouths, and imitate finger movements. Hwang discovered that when a mother's nipple is touched, the prolactin level in her baby increases four to six times. Lee Salk showed that most mothers hold their babies on their left side, and that when babies are held on this side they naturally quiet down to the beating of their mother's heart. Lind investigated the baby's cry and found a significant increase in the amount of blood flow to the mother's breast when she hears her baby's cry.

All of this research has been extremely important for professionals who work with newborns and new parents. However, until recently, the information was not getting to the parents, who so desperately needed it. Concerned with their problem, Dr. Joseph Butterfield of Children's Hospital in Denver gathered persons involved in the research and together they presented their information to health professionals at an important and exciting workshop in Keystone, Colorado. Dr. Butterfield, long sensitive to the needs of parents in crisis, designed the workshop specifically to get the research information into the hands of those who could pass it on to new parents.

Among those present at this workshop were important and caring professionals who wished to share what information they had. Dr. T. Berry Brazelton presented his "Neonatal Behavioral Assessment Scale," the first study that demonstrated the amazing capabilities a newborn brings to her relationship with her parents. With humor and sympathy, he described the needs of new parents to see their infant as an individual person. He described the skills parents need for soothing and playing with their newborn. Dr. Marshall Klaus, who had done important work on infant/maternal bonding and its implication for the family, also shared his work with us. Dr. Doug Pugh, a neonatologist at the University of Colorado Medical Center, gave us the final inspiration and assistance we needed to develop this material into a book that would help new parents.

The common practice of using the pronoun "he" when speaking or writing about the baby to be born or the baby already born is unrealistic and misleading. This inadvertently sets up pregnant parents to expect boys at birth and ignores the families who actually have girls. Since approximately half the babies will be girls and the other half boys, we have decided to alternate pronouns in this book: "he" is used in chapters 1, 3, 5, 7, 9, 11, and 13, and "she" in chapters 2, 4, 6, 8, 10, and 12.

1.

The Importance of the Family

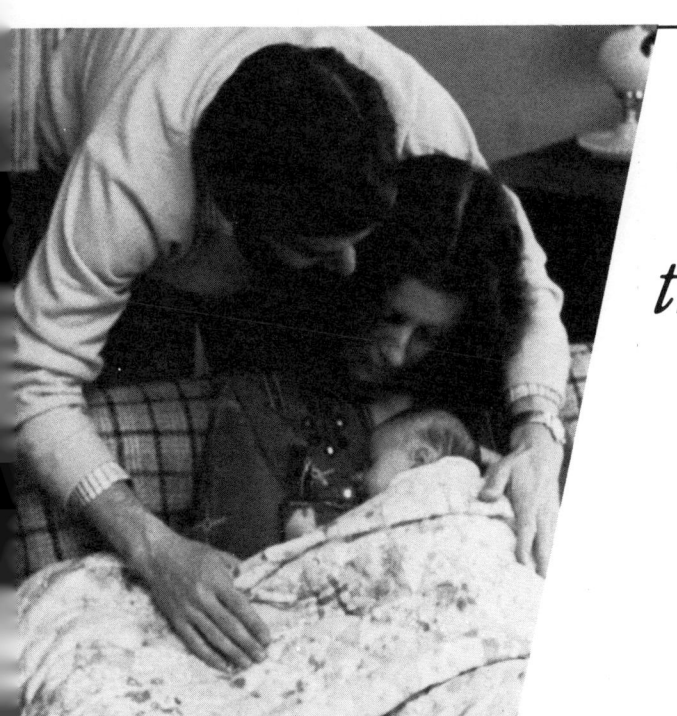

The family unit is the basis of the whole human experience. The concern of human parents for their young is absolutely essential for babies' survival. Human parents are not only involved in the conception, gestation, birth, and care of their newborns, but in a continuing and enduring relationship with their children. As the foundation for every significant society known in the history of humankind, the family has been responsible for preparing the next generation for adult life. The long period of dependence of human children upon their mother and family allows a cultural, social, and emotional inheritance to be passed on that is not possible for any other species.

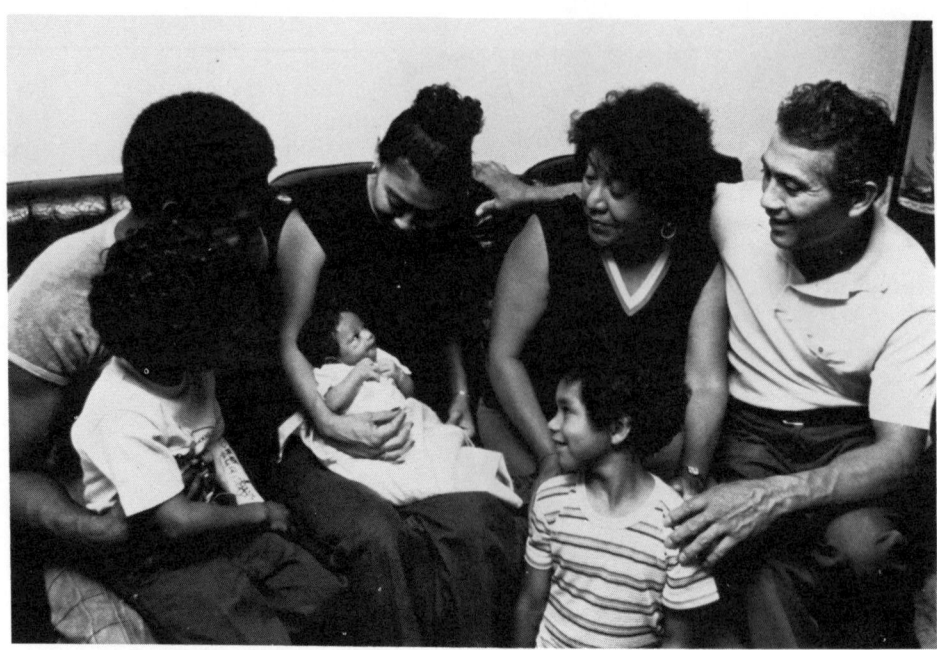

DEVELOPMENT OF THE FAMILY

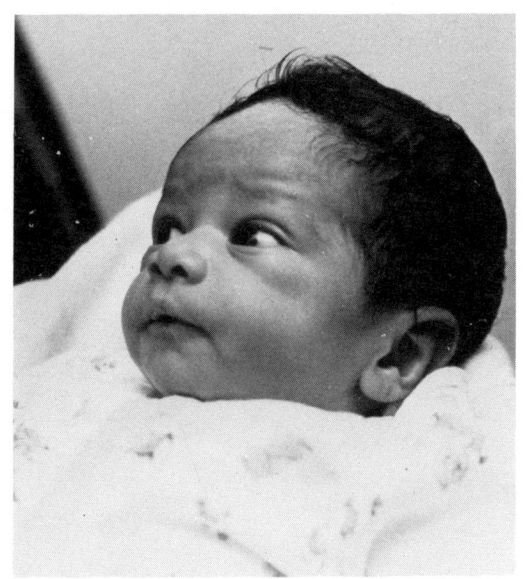

Your family provides a structure that allows your infant to develop a capacity to give and receive love. The family is the most effective institution yet devised to pass on the lessons of tenderness, kindness, and trust. Family bonding creates the loving relationships that make up much of the richness and beauty of life. Until recently the family unit has been thought of as indestructible. We now know that it is a fragile organism that needs confidence, support, and information if it is to survive. Events during pregnancy, birth, and the first days of life form the blueprints for the way the family will integrate this new life and pass on the lessons of love.

Life's most important events—birth and death—have traditionally taken place in the home, surrounded by family. In the past, it was the extended family that supplied vital information and support during pregnancy and birth. Birth and parenting were shared experiences in which a child participated from a very early age.

The development of a more mobile society and hospital births diminished this sharing. Parents were left to cope virtually alone with the profound changes that accompany pregnancy and the birth of an infant. Today, in isolated nuclear families, future parents often have had no exposure to others' experiences of pregnancy, childbirth, or parenting. As they become aware of the profound responsibilities of parenting a newborn, they find that they must seek information and support from sources outside the family.

THE NEWBORN

It was not long ago that mothers and fathers were handed their babies with the understanding that a child was a piece of clay waiting to be molded. Parents were told their infant had few instincts and capabilities and little ability to hear, see, feel, and taste. Parents felt totally responsible for the successful development of their babies, and feared that each word and action would either make or ruin their baby's personality.

Overwhelmed with this awesome task, parents were afraid to follow their own intuition and they turned to experts, who had many ready answers. A generation of parents wracked by guilt was the result. "Where did I go wrong?" was a familiar wail.

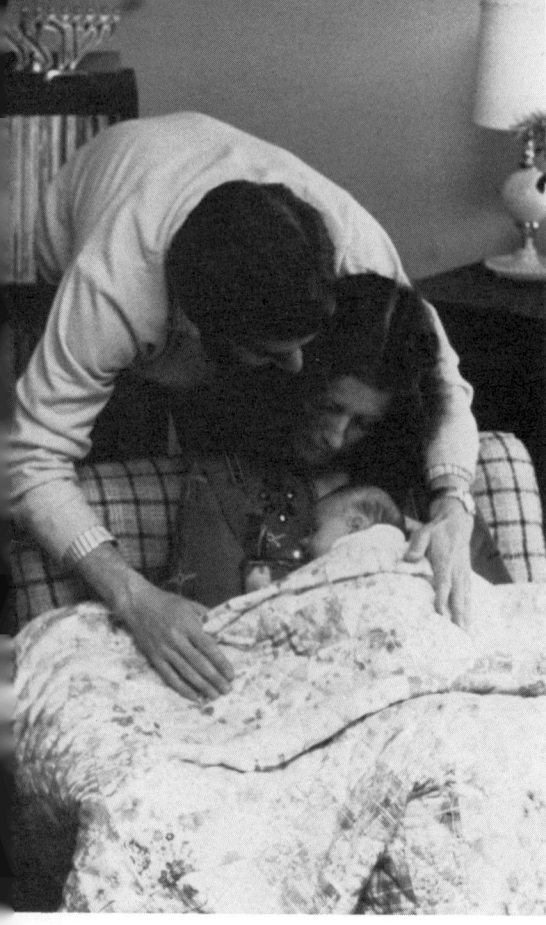

New research has shown us what parents for many past generations have known all along: It takes both the parents and the child to make a relationship. Your baby comes to you with a personality and style all his own that affects your relationship with him. Although you cannot make or break your child, you can help shape your baby by appreciating him or her as a unique individual.

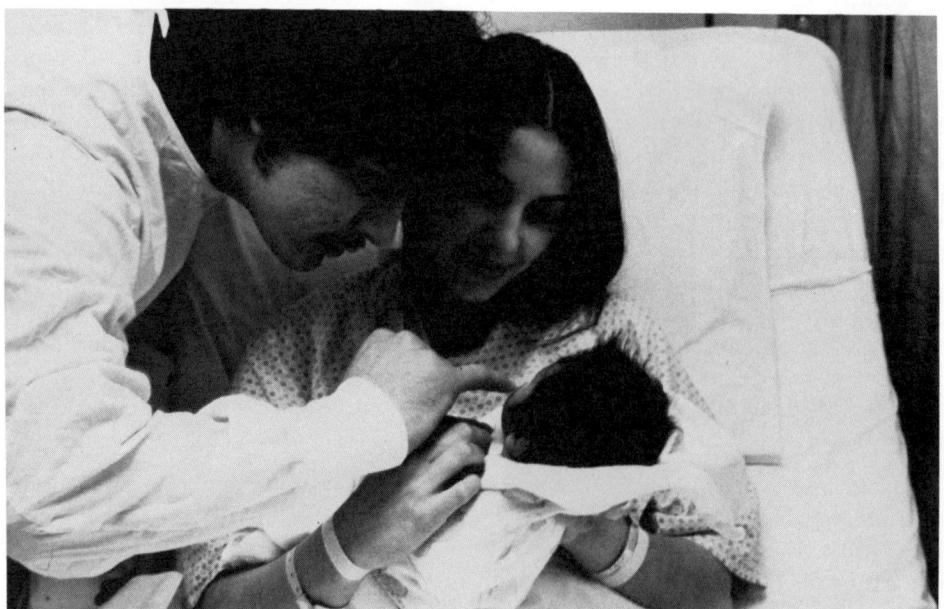

2.

What Kind of Parent Will You Be?

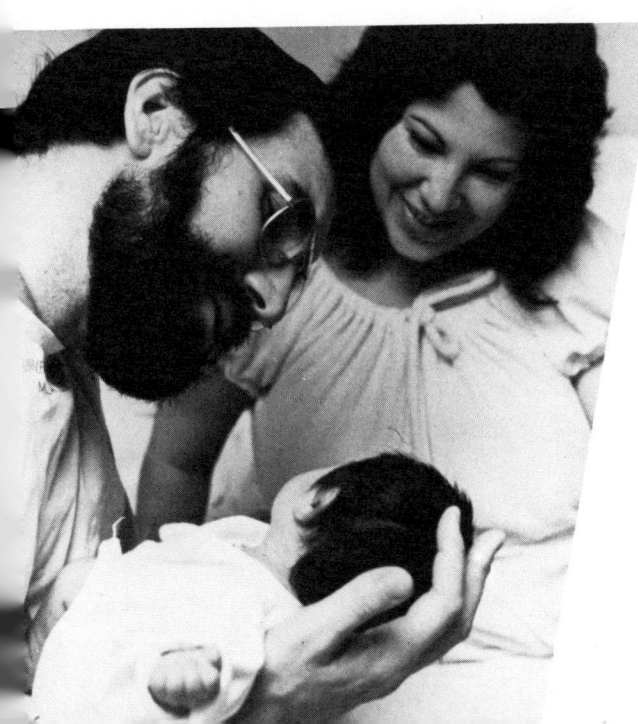

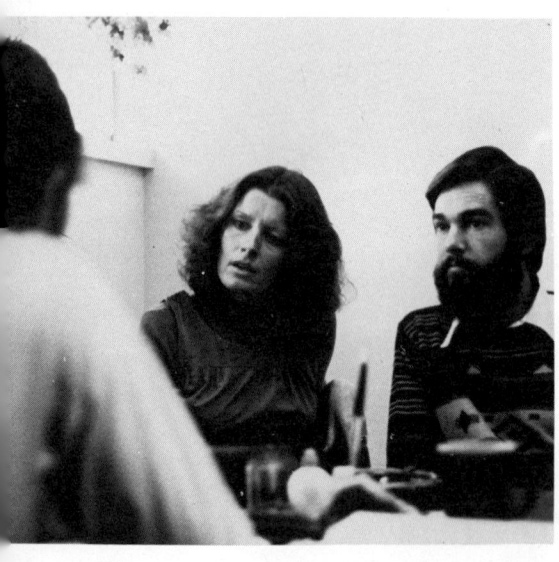

"What kind of a parent will I be?" is a question most expectant parents ask themselves. Although no one can know for sure, we can identify some major factors that influence how you parent.

First, your personality and how you were parented has a significant effect on how you will parent your own baby. Second, we know that the process of parenting the newborn is enhanced when you are active participants in the birth and when you can be together with the baby the first hours after birth. And third, your baby's unique personality and style will help shape your parenting.

PARENTS: YOUR PERSONALITY AND EXPERIENCES

The factors that shape your parenting style are your own personality, your experience of having been parented, your relationships with members of your family, your relationship with your spouse, and your experience with this and previous pregnancies and births.

Self-Esteem

Each person is born with inherited characteristics that are continually modified by life experiences. These experiences influence your perception and understanding of both yourself and the world. Your self-esteem, your ability to handle stress, and your need for attention are essential parts of your personality.

Level of Anxiety

Your level of anxiety and the financial situation surrounding birth, as well as the sex of your baby and order of birth in the family, are also known to affect parenting. The amount of knowledge and preparation you have for pregnancy, childbirth, and parenting is a significant factor in your approach to and enjoyment of parenthood.

How You Were Parented

How you were parented is a good indicator of how you will parent your own children. You will naturally pass on the practices and values of your own family. When you become a parent, both you and your parents will probably relive memories of your childhood. These memories will form the basis of how you will parent your own children. If you are dissatisfied with some of the ways in which you were parented, you can consciously choose a style you think would be better for your own children.

You may become aware of your family heritage for the first time. Your child can bring new richness to the lives of your baby's grandparents and many times brings both new parents a better understanding of and appreciation for their own mothers and fathers.

Pregnancy

During pregnancy and childbirth you, the mother, experience not only a changing body and emotions, but changing roles as well. Your experience with this and previous pregnancies and births influences how you parent this baby. A healthy pregnancy that is wanted and desired, with few major discomforts or problems, helps to enhance parenthood.

Pregnancy and childbirth are often times of emotional crisis for you, the father. You will need to reevaluate your many roles: as a provider for your family, as a father adjusting to the responsibility of this baby, and as a major support for your wife.

Your Marriage

Parenting is also affected by the strength of your marriage relationship. Pregnancy may take place at a time when you, as a couple, are developing an identity of your own. Success in early marriage depends a great deal on the degree of stress you face and your ability to cope with it. Pregnancy and childbirth are clearly stressful times for a couple. The whole structure of your marriage is changed by having a child, especially if it occurs before you have adjusted to adulthood and marriage. On the other hand, the shared act of

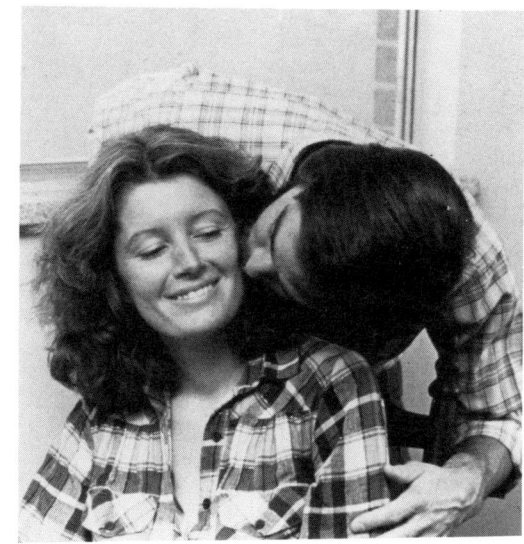

conception and pregnancy can strengthen a marriage and deepen the relationship between you and your partner.

Pregnancy is an important time to improve your communication skills and to become comfortable in expressing your needs and concerns to your partner. The unfamiliar, sometimes frightening changes that pregnancy and parenting bring to your lives may leave both of you upset and frustrated. Establishing more open communication can bring new understanding and appreciation to your marriage.

SUPPORT SYSTEMS

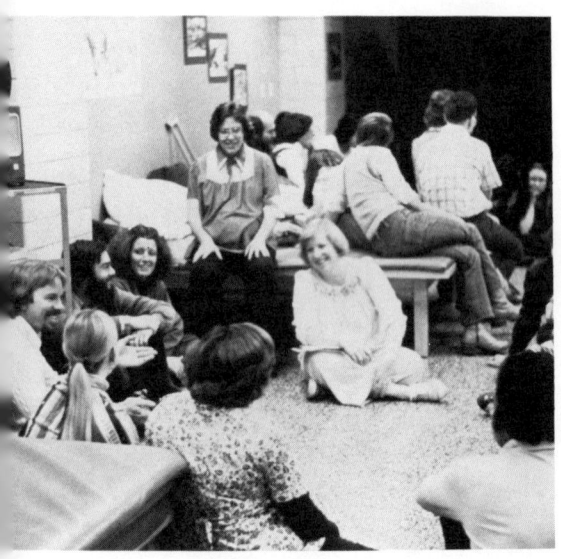

Marriage was never intended to satisfy all the emotional needs of each partner. Pregnancy and childbirth are a special time to expand your support systems. Your extended family can be an important source of support during this period. All the members of your family will be affected by your pregnancy, and how you include them in your preparation for the new baby will greatly influence how the baby is incorporated into your extended family.

Support can come from other sources also: friends, neighbors, religious groups, Red Cross, community nurses, clinics, clubs, and schools. With the increase in nuclear families, special childbirth and parenting groups have assumed the traditional tasks of the extended family in transmitting information, skills, and techniques.

Parenting classes offer accurate and realistic information on the skills needed for feeding, bathing, and caring for your newborn's physical needs. These classes can also help you in the important skills of soothing and playing with your baby. An important part of such classes is the sharing of problems, hopes, and expectations with other mothers and fathers.

BIRTH AND THE FIRST HOURS OF LIFE

We are only now beginning to realize the significance of the second major component of parenting: birth and the first hours of life. There is new and exciting evidence showing that a baby develops a real relationship with her parents in the first hours and days after birth.

Two pioneers in the field of parenting, Dr. Marshall Klaus and Dr. John Kennell, have traced the development of attachment and described how bonds between parent and infant are established. Their work and that of others suggests that maternity care that allows early and extended contact between you and your baby facilitates bonding. If a mother has contact for one hour immediately after birth there may be far-reaching implications, even for a child's later learning and language development.

This new understanding has provided the impetus for developing family-centered maternity care, which provides an atmosphere and facilities that foster the development of warm and loving feelings between you, the parents, and your newborn. Increasingly throughout the United States, hospital practices and policies that inhibit the bonding process have been changed. Enlightened obstetricians, family doctors, midwives, and obstetrical nurses and assistants are all joining forces to ensure the couple privacy and dignity in their birth experience. For normal, uncomplicated labors and births, mothers and fathers are prepared to be active participants. The father is part of the team in the labor and delivery room.

Labor

Labor is a special time in the process of parenting. Attachment is enhanced when parents approach labor with the confidence, knowledge, and skill that allow them to feel in control of the events surrounding the birth experience. The mother emerges from it feeling good about herself, her baby, and her partner. The father not only knows he was an active participant in comforting and assisting with the birth, but admires the new strengths he sees in his wife.

Delivery

Attachment is enhanced when you are awake, alert, and active participants in the delivery of your child. The birth itself, for most prepared parents, is a peak experience and is usually followed by a period of unreserved ecstasy. It is an emotional time when feelings of relief and joy predominate.

SKIN-TO-SKIN CONTACT

Immediately after birth the bonding process begins when your baby is handed to you for skin-to-skin contact. There is no separation from the baby for either the mother or the father. Privacy is given to you to share this time.

EARLY BREAST-FEEDING

If you wish to breast-feed, your baby is put to your breast to nuzzle, root, and lick. Although she might not actually nurse at this time, her action starts the processes that help to ensure successful breast-feeding. Because visual contact is so important, antibiotics or silver nitrate are not put into your baby's eyes for at least an hour.

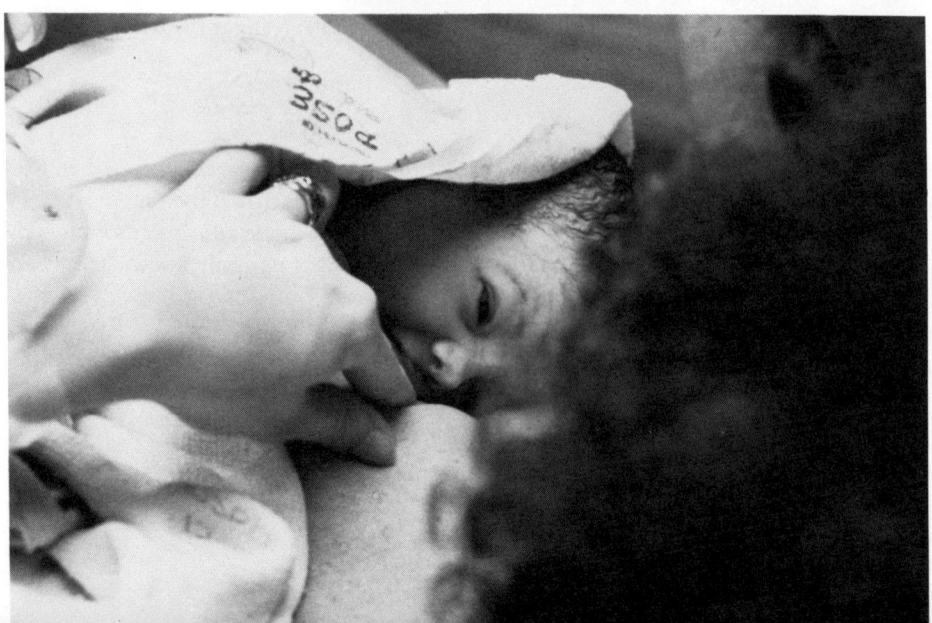

INTERACTIONS

During the first minutes and hours after birth, interactions between mother and baby foster attachment. Mutual touching, eye-to-eye contact, voice—even body heat and odor—are pleasurable to both you and your baby.

Awake and alert, your baby gazes at you and follows your movements with great interest. As she licks your nipple, she sets in motion a physical reaction in which the secretion of the hormone oxytocin into your bloodstream causes your uterus to contract, thereby reducing your postpartum bleeding. Another hormone, prolactin, is also released. It is responsible for promoting the production of milk and is also associated with the mothering and protecting responses. The early transfer of your bacteria to your infant by skin-to-skin contact immunizes her to the bacteria she will encounter in her early months.

During this sensitive period immediately after birth the baby and parents are especially open to the interaction that helps form bonds of attachment. A special interchange takes place among mother, father, and infant. Slow-motion movies show that the baby moves in rhythm to her mother's voice.

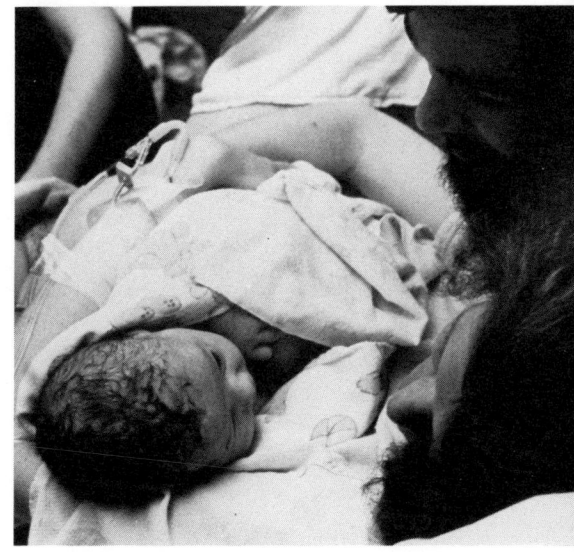

FLEXIBILITY

Bonding is a process that begins before birth and continues throughout a lifetime. It is not limited to a critical period in the first hours and days after birth. Although it seems that early bonds significantly strengthen parent/infant relationships, the flexibility of human nature allows parents who for some reason may miss the sensitive period to overcome the effects of early separation.

BABY: INDIVIDUAL PERSONALITY AND STYLE

The third component of the parenting experience is the personality and style of your baby. Each infant is an individual from the moment of birth, and has her own personality made up of her genetic inheritance from each parent; her own experiences in the uterus; and her birth experience.

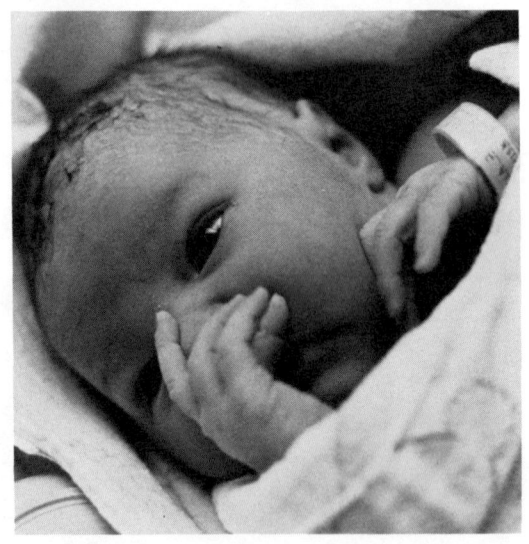

It is important to accept your baby as an individual with a distinct personality, capabilities, and needs. Getting to know your baby is a challenge. Consider her a partner in your relationship and listen to what she can and will tell you.

From the moment of birth, your newborn has the ability to signal her need for care and to initiate pleasurable activity with you. She can guide and reward her parents. Some babies signal more clearly than others, but whatever characteristics your baby has, you will be able to enjoy her if you watch for and listen to her cues as you explore and discover her unique personality.

Some babies are more active than others; some are more regular and predictable in their behavior. Some are delighted with new situations, others upset by changes. Some stay alert for long periods of time, others only for short periods. Some babies cry more and longer and are less easily soothed; others cry less and are easily comforted. Babies also vary in their preferences for kinds of amusement and comfort.

Two babies born on the same day may not be the same physical age at birth. Premature babies may miss out on valuable time for prenatal growth and development. A full-term newborn is stronger and has a more fully developed nervous system for coping with changes.

3.

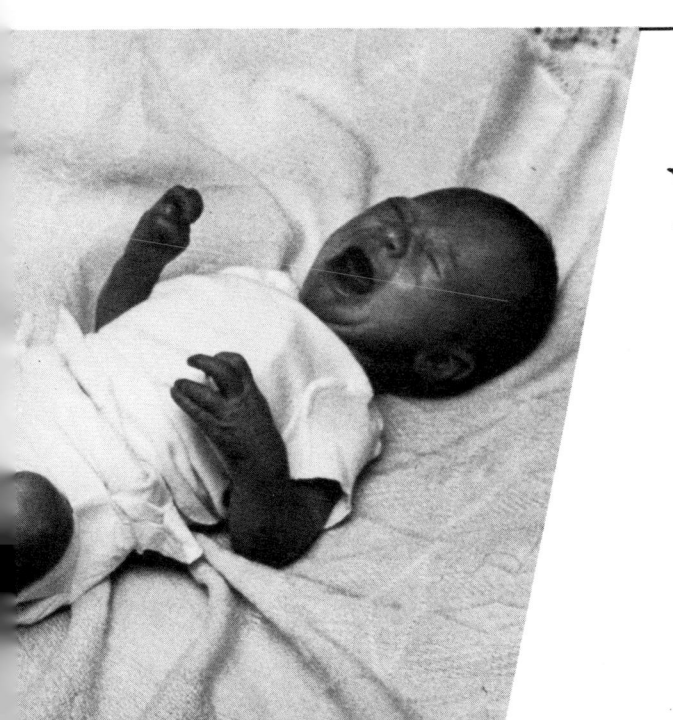

Your Newborn

When your baby is placed in your arms, perhaps the first baby you've ever cared for, you may find that he is very different from what you had anticipated. You may have some anxious moments because, even though society expects you to acquire the skills of a mother spontaneously, being a parent is actually a learned role.

BIRTH

Since your baby may swallow mucus and fluids during his journey down the birth canal, the doctor suctions his nose and mouth. When he takes his first breath, his heart begins to pump blood for the first time through his lungs. He begins to breathe; his color improves.

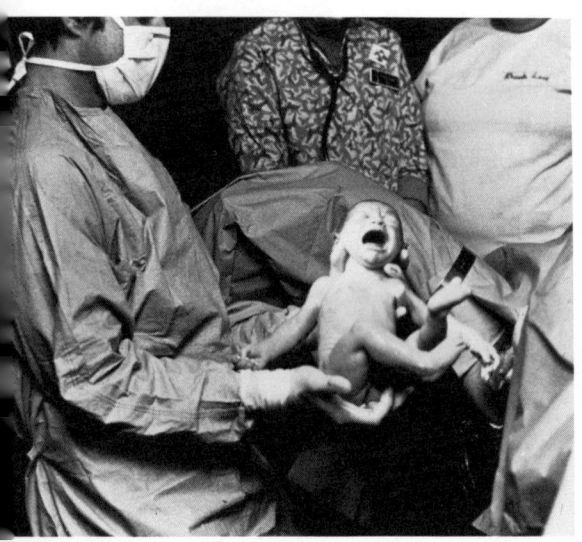

Cutting the Cord

When circulation is cut off to the umbilical cord, the doctor clamps it in two places, a few inches apart. The first clamp is placed a few inches from your baby's abdomen. Then the cord is cut between the clamps and your baby is placed on your abdomen. The other segment of the cord is still attached to your placenta and is delivered when the placenta is expelled.

First Breath

As your newborn is delivered, the rapid expansion of his chest, the abrupt change from fluid to air, and the drop in temperature of his environment cause his lungs to open. Many newborns breathe as soon as the head is delivered. Since your baby has not breathed on his own before, but has received his oxygen supply from you, his first breaths are the most difficult and the most critical. Newborns' breathing may be quite irregular and inconsistent.

APGAR Scale

To evaluate your baby's condition, the doctor or nurse uses the APGAR scale, which notes quality of skin color, ability to breathe, heart rate, muscle tone, and reflex irritability at birth. A baby born with a uniform skin tone, a strong cry, a heart rate of more than 100, and good active muscle tone is evaluated at 10. Babies receiving scores of 7 or under are taken to the nursery for close observation. It's not unusual for many babies' fingers and toes to be bluish immediately after birth. An APGAR scale evaluation of 8 or more is generally a sign of a healthy baby.

APGAR Scoring Chart

sign	0	1	2
heart rate	absent	slow (below 100)	over 100
respiratory effort	absent	weak cry, hypoventilation	good strong cry
muscle tone	limp	some flexion of extremities	well flexed
reflex response	no response	grimace	cough or sneeze cry and withdrawal of foot
color	blue, pale	body pink extremities blue	completely pink

Weighing and Measuring

Healthy, full-term babies usually measure 18–20 inches and weigh about 7–8 pounds. They may lose a few ounces the first few days after birth, but regain them within the first two weeks.

Body Temperature

Your baby does not have the resources to counter the effects of either heat or cold. Many doctors believe that skin-to-skin contact with your body is the best way to maintain your baby's body temperature, in addition to being an effective way to facilitate the bonding process.

Identification

While you are still in the delivery room, two identical identification bands are secured on your baby's wrist and ankle. The bands describe the sex of your baby, your full name and hospital admission number, and the date and time of birth. An identical band is made for you and placed on your wrist. Your baby's footprints and your right index fingerprint are recorded on your baby's hospital record.

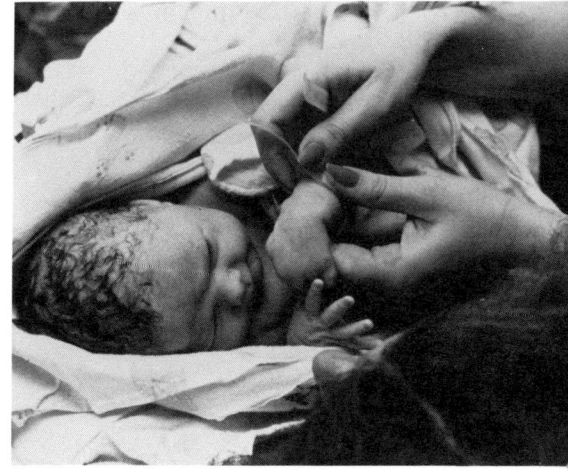

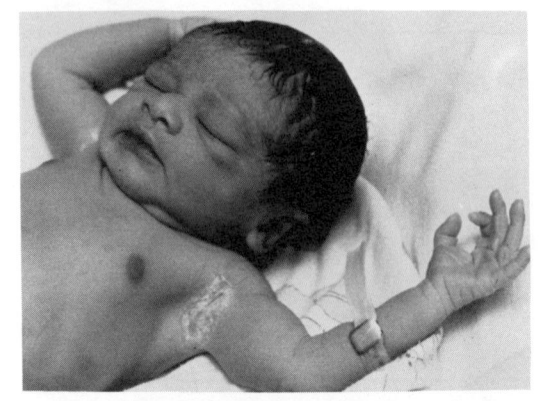

PHYSICAL CHARACTERISTICS

Skin

A creamy white substance called the vernix caseosa covers your baby to protect his skin in the uterus. After birth, the vernix is absorbed into the skin and usually disappears within twenty-four hours. Your baby's skin may be discolored, or wrinkled and loose, or scaly in creased places, such as hands and feet. Some newborns have extra stores of flesh, part of which is fluid, that make them look fat. This condition helps to tide over your newborn until he can eat. As the extra padding disappears during the first week, it may leave the skin peeled and cracked.

Hair

Besides the hair on his head, dark, fine hair called lanugo may be present on your baby's body. The hair, matted with vernix, can give him a strange pasted look. The lanugo disappears by about the fourth week, leaving your baby soft and smooth.

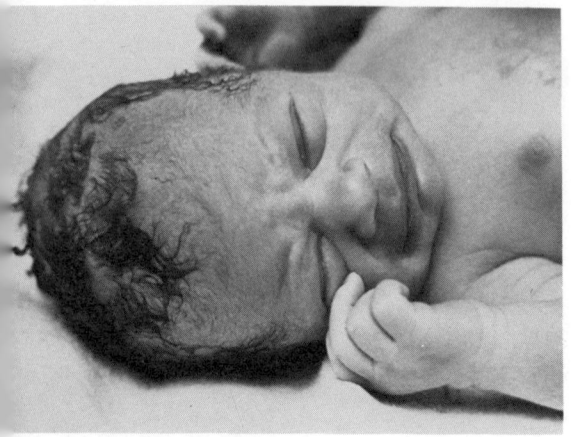

Head

For the first day or so, your baby's head may be swollen at the top because of the pressure against your pelvic outlet during birth. Since your baby's head is almost one-third of his height and an inch larger in diameter than his chest, his movements are awkward. The anterior fontanel, or soft spot, can be felt on top of his head. The fontanel on the back of the head is smaller. Because your baby's neck is not strong enough to support the weight of his head, it wobbles unless you hold it.

Face

His face may be puffy and bluish, and his ears pressed to his head. His eyelids appear puffy and may even be bruised. In a few days these all become normal. His nose, flattened by passage through the birth canal, soon resumes its normal shape. Mucus may be present in his nostrils. His lips are pinkish and will begin sucking when touched. Small white spots may be seen on the gum margins.

Eyes

Your newborn's eyes are slate blue or gray. It usually takes several months for the eyes to attain their permanent color. Uncoordinated eye movements are normal. Some state laws require that silver nitrate or an antibiotic be placed in your baby's eyes to prevent blindness caused by gonorrhea or syphilis. Application of drops may be delayed to facilitate the eye contact so important to the attachment process.

Abdomen

His abdomen is rounded and prominent. The umbilical stump dries within several hours after birth. An umbilical hernia may be present, but it is usually insignificant.

Genitals

Because of the hormones secreted during pregnancy, and the stresses of labor and delivery, your baby's genitals may appear enlarged. If you have a girl, the lips of her vulva may be swollen. There may even be a little spotting of blood from her vagina. If you have a boy, his scrotum may be swollen. In both boys and girls, hormones may cause a swelling of the breasts.

Bowel Movements

Your baby's first bowel movements are of a brownish-green soft material called meconium. It is made up of cast-off cells and swallowed amniotic fluid. After the third or fourth day, the meconium is replaced by light yellow feces. For the first few days solid stools are not formed. Your newborn eliminates a large amount of urine, feces, and sweat, which causes a temporary weight loss.

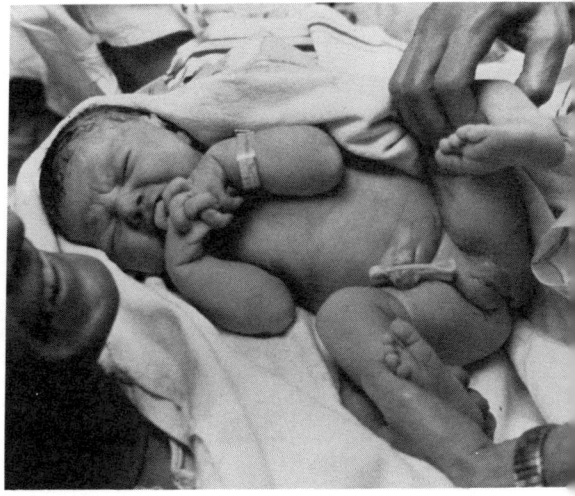

Jaundice

After babies are born, some of their red blood cells break down and form a substance called bilirubin, which is then processed by the liver for elimination. Some babies whose livers are immature cannot assimilate these waste products fast enough. The excess of wastes builds up in their bodies, causing a yellow tint in the skin and the whites of their eyes. This condition is known as jaundice. About one-third of all newborns become visibly jaundiced between the second and fifth day of life. Usually this condition begins to clear up after three days.

Breathing

Your newborn's rate of breathing, 36 to 48 breaths per minute, is twice as fast as yours. It is quite irregular, full of starts and stops, snorts, hiccups, gaggings, sneezes, coughs, and gasps. He may have swallowed a lot of mucus during his journey through the birth canal and may have to clear his breathing passages.

Sleep

Soon after delivery, your baby relaxes and falls into a deep, comalike sleep. A brief change in breathing is the only response to loud noise. At this time, your baby is taken to the nursery, where nurses observe his breathing, check his cardiovascular system, and maintain his temperature. The first day of life is a critical one.

SENSORY ABILITIES

In your uterus your baby could see, hear, touch, and taste. From the moment of birth these senses help him deal with his environment, letting him express satisfaction and displeasure and fostering his interactions with you.

Sight

Your newborn can focus his eyes at birth, but the most exciting discovery is that he prefers the human face and can make eye contact with you. On the delivery table, he can turn to your face and gaze into your eyes. He sees best at a distance of eight to twelve inches, just the distance from your face when you hold him in your arms. Your newborn can distinguish light from dark and prefers bright colors, movements, and simple shapes and patterns. When he becomes alert to your face as an object, he stares intently, his eyes shining with interest. His face brightens and his body motions quiet down. If an object is moved slowly from side to side he can usually follow it with his eyes and turn his head slowly with the movements. He can even follow the object up and down. His movements are not very smooth until three to six weeks after birth.

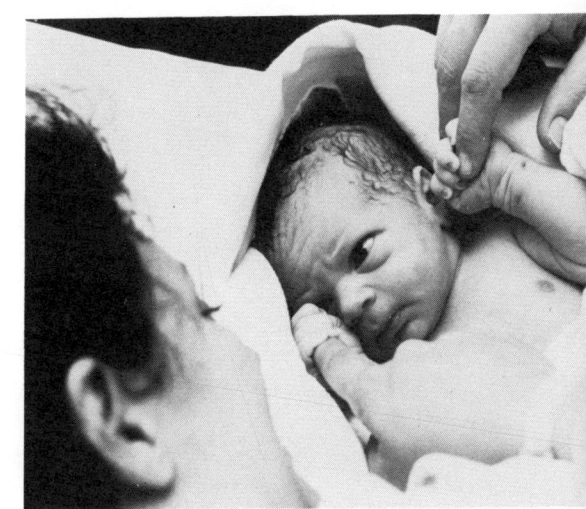

Hearing

Your baby is not only born with the ability to hear, but he actually enjoys and prefers certain sounds. While in the uterus your newborn hears your heartbeat and digestive noises and your voice. At birth, your baby hears and turns toward a human voice, but likes one that is high-pitched rather than low. Fathers find themselves talking in a falsetto to get the attention of their baby. When your baby listens to your speech, he moves his arms and legs in slow motion with your speech patterns. Soft, pleasant, rhythmic noises, like crooning or humming, are soothing to your baby.

Touch

Your newborn is very sensitive to touch and pressure. Skin contact and warmth from your body are your baby's most powerful stimulation. He can sense and respond to comforting, soothing handling. Your baby prefers a warm and gentle touch and responds to rhythmic stroking and rocking. He withdraws from painful stimuli such as excessive heat, cold, and pressure.

Taste

When your baby is born he can distinguish between sweet, sour, bitter, and salty tastes, and shows a preference for sweet and a dislike of bitter flavors. He prefers human milk, which is sweeter than cow's milk or formula.

Smell

Your baby's sense of smell is already developed. He can differentiate between smells, and can distinguish the odor of his mother when he is five days old.

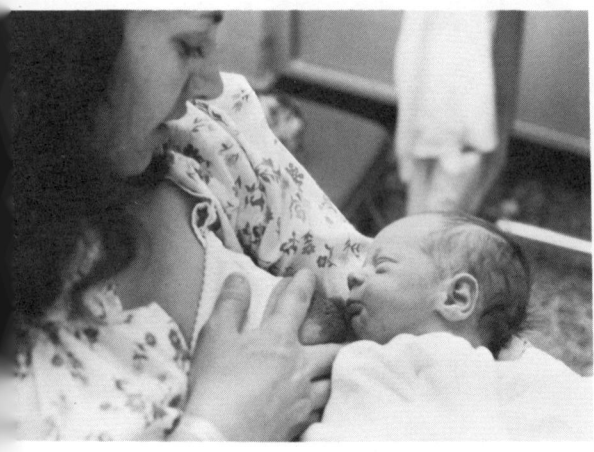

THE FIRST DAYS OF LIFE

During the first few days, your baby is recovering from labor, delivery, and the initial stresses of life outside the uterus. His job is to stabilize his circulation, breathing, digestion, elimination, body temperature, and hormone mechanisms, which must work faster for his new life. This self-reorganization, however, leaves little energy for eating and digesting. Many babies don't care to eat at all. During your baby's first few days, he cannot digest even milk. His stores of extra sugar, fat, and fluid sustain him until your milk comes in.

Prior to birth, your body provided a constant environment for your baby. Now the newborn must digest his own food, regulate his own body temperature in an inconstant climate, and breathe in order to secure oxygen. He may urinate as much as 18 times daily and move his bowels 4–7 times. He sleeps 14–18 hours of the day. On the average, he is alert for only 30 minutes in a four-hour period.

The early hours and days are your time to get to know your baby as an individual. Take time to undress and examine his body. Become accustomed to his special features. Listen to his cry. Pay special attention to him when he is quiet and awake. Although his immature nervous system does not yet give him control over his reactions, it is fun to look for those things that soothe and give him pleasure.

Reflexes

Your baby is born with reflexes that help him control his environment. Sucking and swallowing are important for survival. Blinking, sneezing, coughing, and withdrawing help protect him. Other reflexes are forerunners of skills your baby will develop as he matures.

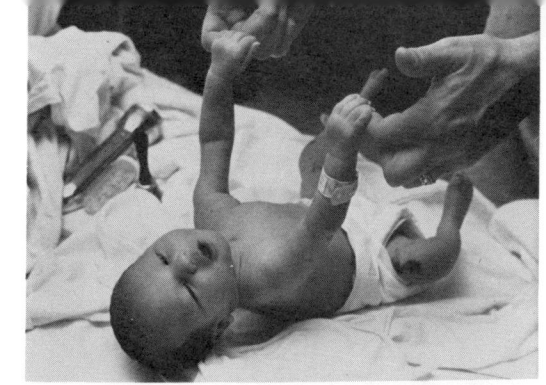

PROTECTION REFLEXES

The blink reflex keeps annoying matter or too much light out of your baby's eyes. The sneezing reflex clears out his nasal passages, and the coughing reflex helps him clear his throat. If his breathing is interfered with, he can turn his head to clear his face. He blinks, sneezes, stretches, burps, hiccups, twitches and has jerky movements. All are normal and common.

GRASP REFLEX

Your baby is born with a grasp reflex in both his hands and feet. He will grasp a finger (or any other object) placed in his palm. This reflex not only helps him hold on to his mother, giving him a feeling of safety and a sense of security, but also gives you a feeling of closeness. His hand grasp is so strong that you can gently pull him to a sitting position.

STANDING REFLEX

When a newborn is placed in a standing position, he flexes his legs underneath his body and places his weight on them.

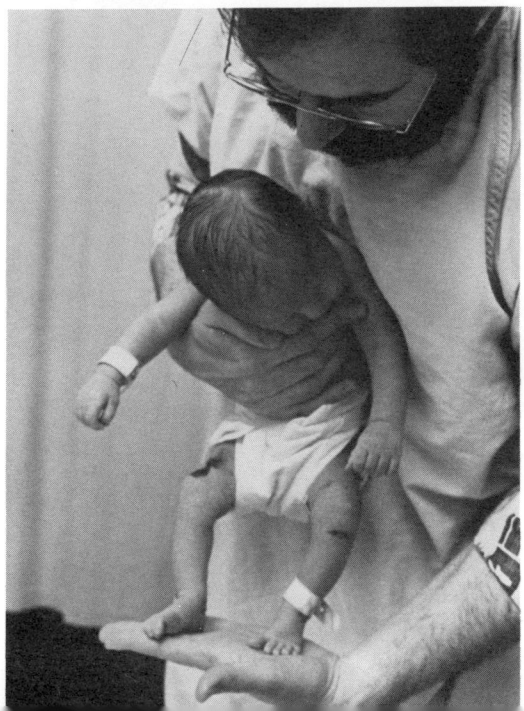

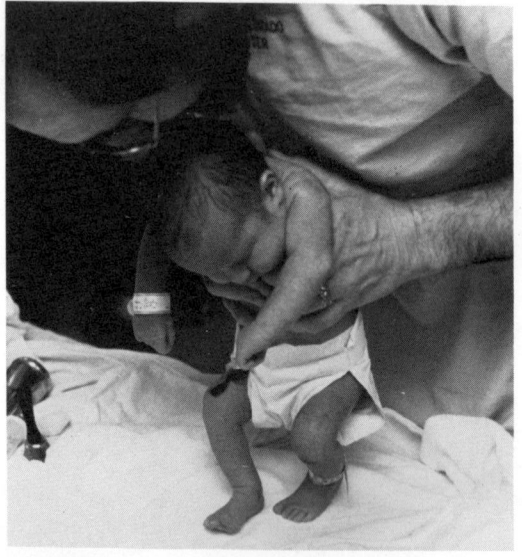

WALKING REFLEX

When you hold your newborn in this position and lean him forward, he will automatically stand on one leg and begin to move the other leg in front of him. This reflex, a precursor to walking, usually disappears around eight weeks of age.

PLACING REFLEX

When you stroke or tap the bottom of your baby's hand or foot, it will stretch out, cover your hand, and grasp your finger. This may be an evolutionary development, since primates have the same reflex ability. If the foot or hand of a baby monkey hits the limb of a tree, this reflex allows it to catch the limb to keep from falling.

CRAWLING/SWIMMING REFLEX

Long before birth, your baby was an accomplished swimmer in your uterus. Like any amphibian, he could rhythmically extend his arms and legs, swing his trunk from side to side, and stop breathing for periods in the uterus. This movement will soon be used for the important development of crawling.

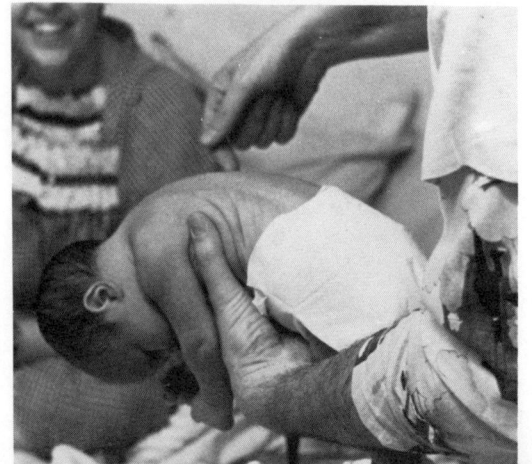

INCURVATURE REFLEX

Human beings have easily distinguishable right and left sides, with most organs and appendages arranged in pairs. The central nervous system lies along the dorsal, or back, side of our bodies, a characteristic that evolved with the primitive fishes more than 400 million years ago. When you support your baby on his stomach and stroke the muscles along one side of his backbone, he will turn his pelvis toward the side stimulated, signaling that his nervous system is functioning properly.

RIGHTING REFLEX

Your baby's head is too heavy for the muscles of his neck and back to support. He is born with a righting reflex intended to keep his head upright. You can see this reflex as he is pulled by his arms from his back to a sitting position. His eyes open wide and his entire shoulder area tenses as he helps to pull up his head. As his head flops forward, he will try to keep it upright, and in that attempt, his head falls backward. General muscle tone affects the response. His head control will improve as his muscle strength increases.

DOLL'S EYE REFLEX

When your baby is pulled to a sitting position or held upright with his body flexed at the waist, his eyes open in a doll's eye reflex. Placing your baby in a sitting position and rocking him from side to side is a good way of getting him to open his eyes and become alert and receptive.

ROOTING REFLEX

As your baby's cheek is touched, he will turn toward the stimulus. When your baby is put to your breast after birth, he turns toward it and begins to search or root for the nipple. This rooting reflex helps your baby locate your nipple, assuring the success of feeding in the newborn period.

SUCKING REFLEX

Once your newborn has rooted for your nipple, he opens his mouth and takes it in, initiating the sucking reflex. The sucking reflex begins once the mucous membranes inside his mouth come in contact with an object. A newborn will often suck his own fist or fingers for long periods; we know that such sucking in the uterus is common.

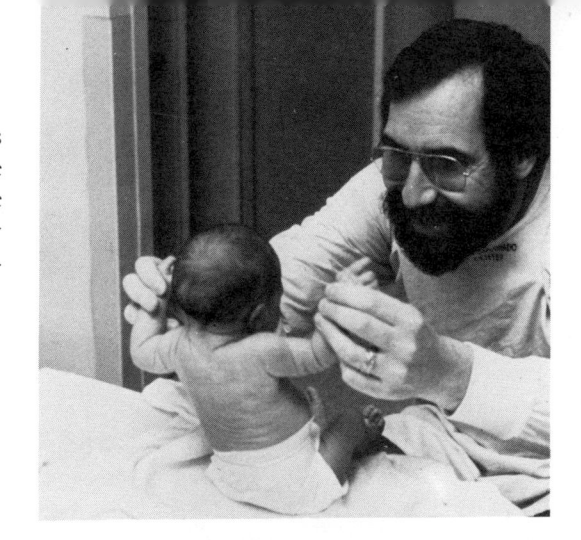

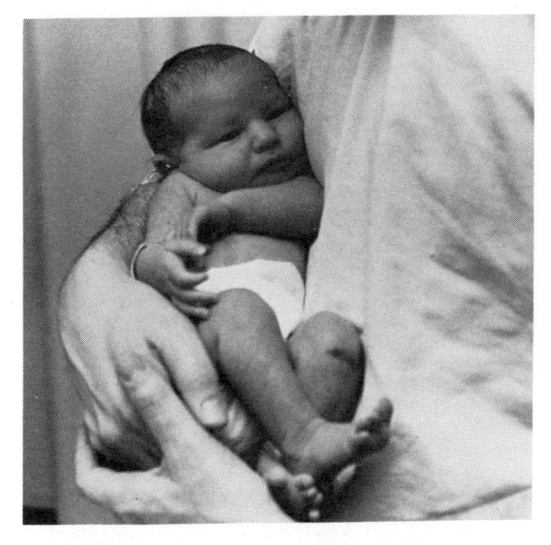

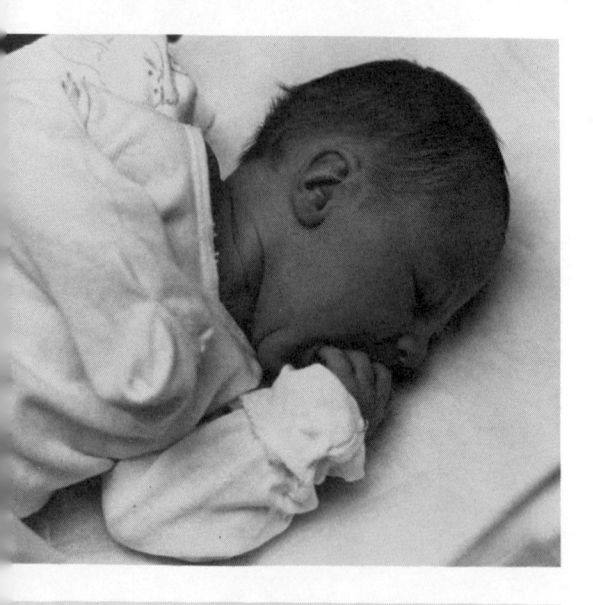

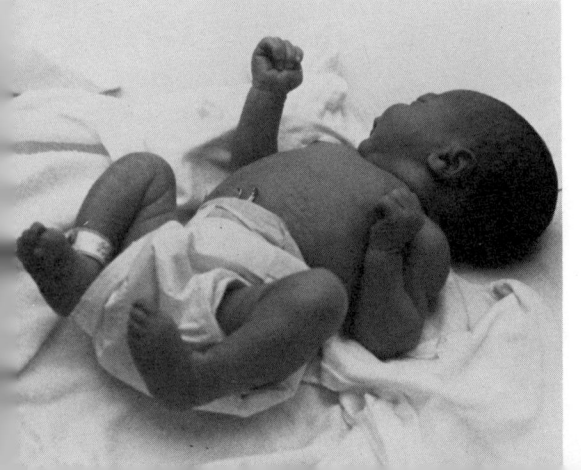

HAND-TO-MOUTH REFLEX

Your baby is born with a hand-to-mouth reflex that helps him soothe himself. When his cheek is stroked, his arms flex, and he may bring his hand up to his mouth and place his fist or fingers in it. This allows him to fulfill his sucking needs for himself.

PROTECTIVE WARMTH REFLEX

One of the most critical physical challenges of a newborn is to maintain his temperature. He will pull his arms and legs in to his body to cut down on the amount of body surface exposed. He cries and shivers to improve circulation and to signal for help. When he is covered and warm, he quiets down.

MOTOR TONE REFLEXES

Whether on his back or stomach, your baby will tend to lie in a curled-up or flexed position, much like his position in the uterus. When the arms or legs are extended away from the body, normal infants have a reflex that brings them back to their natural flexed position. These smooth movements of extension and flexion are called motor tone. When you pick up your baby, his body movement usually responds to you. A limp baby gives little feedback to a parent, and a tense baby with jerky movements can be disconcerting.

SMOTHER REFLEX

Your infant is not helpless. He can avoid smothering with protective reflexes. Placed on his tummy, with his head down, he can pick his head up off the bed and turn it to one side or the other. If a cloth is placed over his nose and mouth, he moves vigorously and twists his head from side to side to escape it.

TONIC NECK REFLEX

When your baby's head is turned to one side or the other, his whole body arches away from the side to which the head is turned. The arm on the face side extends upward, and the other arm flexes in a fencing position. This is called the tonic neck reflex. It helps your baby to learn how to use one side of his body separately from the other.

WITHDRAWAL REFLEX

Because constant stimulation can overwhelm your newborn's immature systems, he is born with mechanisms that help him control his environment. When faced with an annoying stimulus your baby can actively withdraw from it by shrinking, turning away, or arching his body. He can push it away with his hands or feet or withdraw into drowsiness or sleep. If all else fails, he has the power to fuss or cry, which brings a parent to help him deal with the unpleasant stimulus. It is important to notice how your infant withdraws, so that you can respond to these signals of overstimulation.

CUDDLE REFLEX

One of the most important characteristics your baby brings with him is the ability to cuddle. When held, a baby usually nestles into his parent's body. This causes the parents to want to hold him tighter and to cuddle and love him. This active cuddling response makes it easy for new parents to become attached to their baby, but with an infant who is not responsive, the parents are likely to feel rejected. If your baby lies passively or slides through your arms, or if, on the other hand, he resists being held by stiffening up and thrashing about, you will probably feel rejected. It should help you to know that if your baby is a noncuddler, it is not your fault, but only your baby's particular style. It is important to learn your baby's style and let him direct you in finding other ways to feel close.

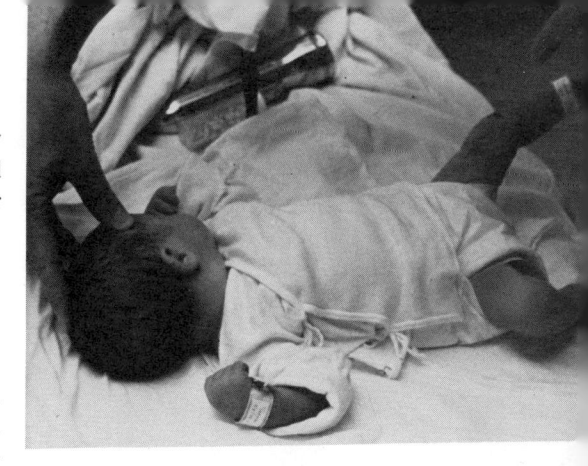

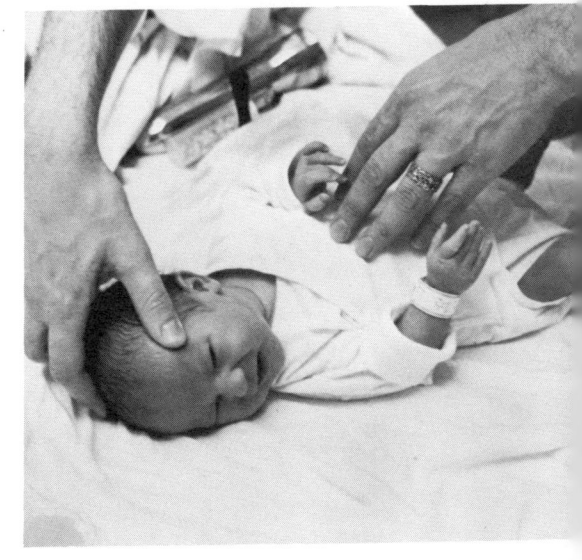

Sleeping and Waking States

Your baby will experience six basic states of waking and sleeping. Each of these states—quiet sleep, active sleep, dozing, alert, fussy, and crying—is significant in the growth and development of your child and affects your interaction with him. Learning to recognize the times when your baby is most responsive to stimulation or consoling helps you match your actions to his needs.

QUIET SLEEP

New babies sleep about 14–18 hours a day, with alternating periods of quiet and active sleep. During deep sleep your newborn breathes regularly with his eyes closed. He shows no activity except for jerky movements at regular intervals. Deep sleep is a time for growth and development.

ACTIVE SLEEP

In active sleep, your baby is more receptive to external stimulation. You may observe whimpers, grimaces, smiles, frowns, and random movements. His breathing is irregular, and sucking motions can be seen. Random eye movements can be observed under his closed eyelids. Active sleep is thought to be a time for absorption and reorganization of stimuli and experiences taken in during waking periods.

DOZING

Between the sleeping and alert state your baby passes through a drowsy or semidozing state. His eyes may be closed or open. Your baby may be waking or falling asleep, and his eyes are dull, glazed, or unfocused with droopy eyelids. There may be mild jerks. If waking, your infant can often be brought to the alert state by placing him in a sitting position against your shoulder. He usually becomes more active before feeding and urination.

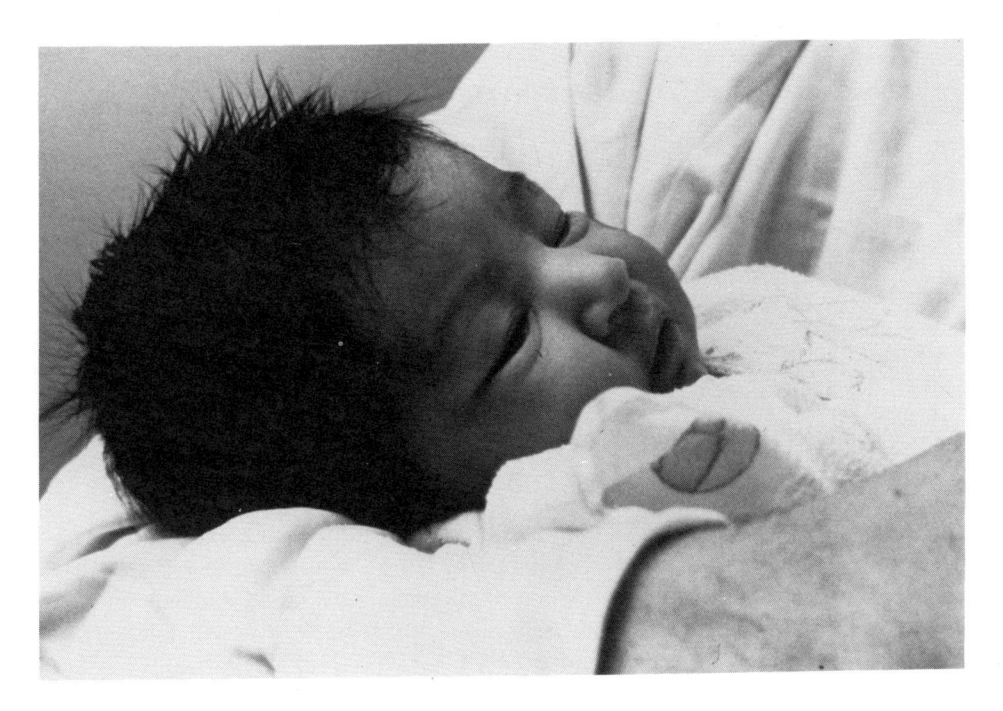

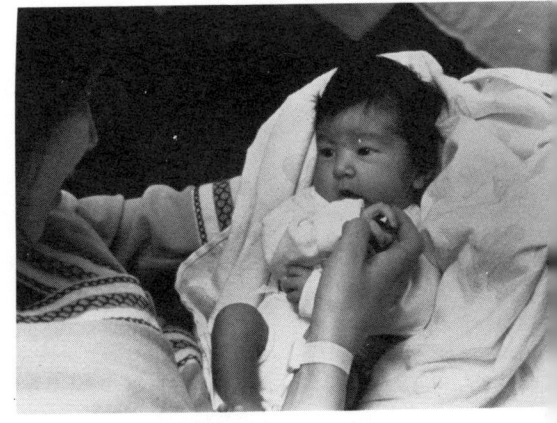

ALERT

The alert awake state is the one in which your baby is most able to receive and process information and respond to you. This is the time when he is most open to change and ready to learn.

A newborn can be alert for as much as an hour or as little as a few minutes every four hours. He is likely to be most responsive to new sights, sounds, and stimulation right after he is fed, changed, and bubbled. His ability to focus his attention is fascinating. When your baby stops moving, focuses on you, and establishes eye contact, you are helping to develop the rhythm and pattern of communication between you.

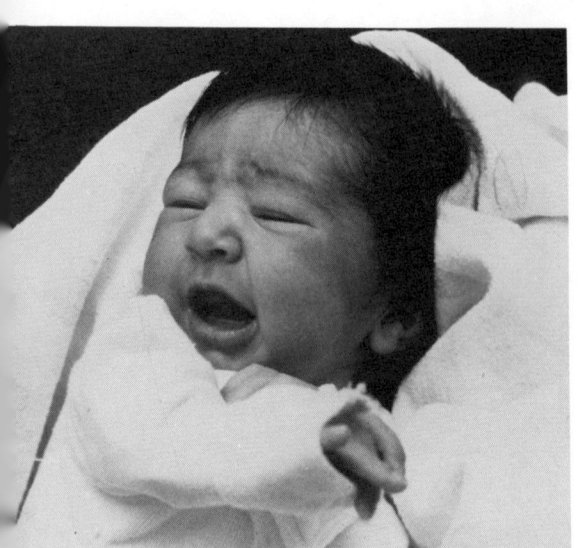

FUSSY

Fussiness or irritability is a positive function in which your baby signals his discomfort or overstimulation. During the state of fussiness, your baby tunes out, turns away, and withdraws his attention. When in this state, he may set up a cycle that makes him more sensitive to annoying stimulation. By soothing and consoling him, you can sometimes interrupt the cycle and bring him back to the alert state, where he is once again ready to take in information.

CRYING

A newborn's cry is one of the most powerful stimuli in the human experience. It signals distress and calls for action. Newborns cry for 20–30 minutes up to 5 times a day. They usually cry before feedings, changings, or sleeping. Babies differ not only in what annoys them, but also in what soothes them. Your baby may cry because he's hungry, in pain, bored, overstimulated, tired, or frustrated.

Because his crying upsets you, your greatest challenge is to respond with soothing behaviors. How your newborn reacts to your consoling efforts greatly affects your feelings about yourself as a mother. If your baby is soothed, you feel rewarded and will probably repeat your efforts. If your baby will not be consoled, you may feel ineffectual and frustrated.

Smiling. Smiling, unlike crying, is not present immediately after birth as a fully developed response system. Your newborn's smiles occur usually during sleep and drowsiness, though there may be some early smiles during wakefulness. Smiles in active sleep appear to be spontaneous behavior coming from within the baby. Social smiling begins at about two months of age, and is readily brought on by a human face.

Behavior Patterns

Your newborn's individual behavior pattern influences the way you react to him. Some mothers have babies who cry little, sleep a lot, are predictable and regular in their schedules, are adaptable and spend a lot of time relating during their waking alert periods. Other mothers have babies who cry a lot, sleep and eat at irregular and unpredictable times, and are less adaptable. These babies may be more difficult to parent and the parents will have to rely on their inner resources to help them meet their baby's needs.

Since parents also have their own particular personalities, a discrepancy may exist between the mother's style and her baby's. A very active mother may be quite disturbed by a passive baby, whereas a passive mother would be quite contented. On the other hand, a very passive mother may be distraught by an active baby. A baby's temperament is part of his personality and cannot be changed, but with understanding and compassion, a mother can work with her baby to develop a mutually satisfying relationship.

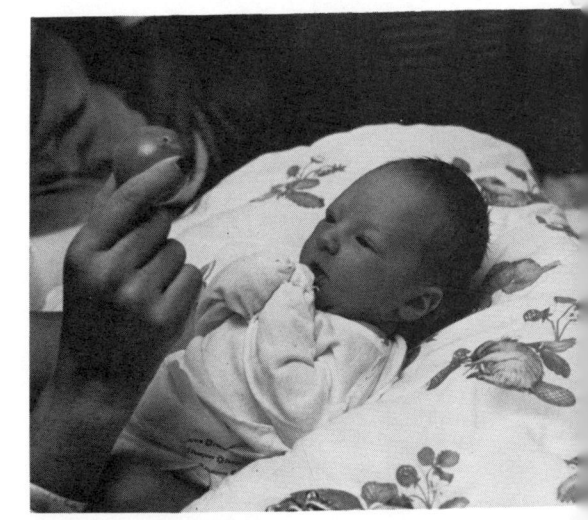

ABILITY TO ENJOY

Visual. Your baby is able to choose and enjoy those things he finds interesting. Babies prefer bright, circular objects. When you show a newborn a red ball, he focuses on it. As the ball is moved slowly from side to side, he will follow it with his eyes. At home, your baby will enjoy colored objects such as mobiles in the crib and colorful wallpaper.

Sounds. Your baby also likes pleasant sounds and shows interest in them. When he hears a bell he will shift his head in its direction. When the bell is rung on the other side, your baby will turn his head all the way around to follow the sound. He will enjoy hearing different kinds of sounds such as rattles and bells.

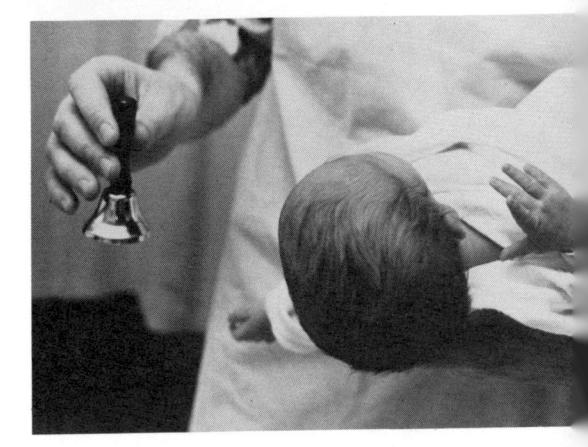

Human face. Your baby loves your face and voice. When you put your face right into his line of vision, he will quiet down and his eyes and face become bright and alert. As you move your face slowly to one side, your baby will usually follow with his eyes and head. Then, when you move it slowly to the other side, he will follow it again. When you play with your baby, there is nothing more interesting than your face. Your baby enjoys focusing on you and gazing into your eyes.

Human voice. Newborns like a variety of pleasant, high-pitched tones. When your baby hears your voice, even if you are out of his line of vision, he will quiet down, his eyes will brighten, and he will shift toward the sound, turning his head. When you move your voice to the other side, your baby will usually follow with his body. Your infant loves to hear your voice and loves you to talk. It does not make any difference what you say; what matters is your voice and its changing, rhythmic tones.

ABILITY TO SHUT OUT ANNOYING STIMULI

One of your infant's most impressive skills is his ability to tune out what he does not want to respond to.

Visual. When a light is shined into a newborn's eyes, the baby will be startled at first, but by the fourth flash he will stop blinking, shut his eyes, and block out the annoying stimulus.

Noise. Your baby can shut out annoying sounds. When a baby hears a bell rung for the first time, he will be startled, but by the third time he will quiet down, stop blinking, and begin to breathe normally. These are adaptive responses that show your baby can protect himself from the noise of the delivery room, nursery, or home. When your baby goes home, the family will not have to go around on tiptoe speaking in hushed tones. It is also important to note that there is a limit to what your baby will take in and be aware of, to avoid being overloaded with stimuli.

CAPACITY TO RESPOND

When you play with your baby, you will begin to notice how easily he is brought into the alert state and how long this state is maintained during your interactions. This gives you some idea of your baby's capacity for responsiveness. Some babies have a long alert period, during which they can tune into the person they are relating with and send and receive messages. These babies give a lot of pleasure to the parent. Some babies have only a short period before they withdraw. They may need more special attention and playtime with their parents to help them develop a longer alert period.

ACTIVITY LEVEL

Some newborns are very active. They move around a lot, kick off covers, squirm and twist. A baby with an extremely high activity level may give his mother no rest. Other babies are calm, quiet, and less active. Still others may remain still in their beds or cribs for long periods of time. Parents might want to cuddle and play with these babies even at times when they don't ask for it.

PREDICTABILITY

Some newborns are very regular in their schedules and predictable in their behavior. They eat every two or three hours, sleep on schedule and even have predictable bowel movements. Others may be erratic in their eating and sleeping schedules, making the mother's planning more difficult. These babies need to be gently pressed into developing regular schedules.

LEVEL OF IRRITABILITY

Each baby not only has his own level of irritability but is irritated by different things. Some babies may be able to shut out many annoying stimuli, and others can cope with only a few.

As you become aware of your baby's sensory level, you can adjust the amount of input he receives, acting as a filter for outside stimuli. Although this is important for all babies, it is critical for those who are unusually irritable or who have a low sensory threshold.

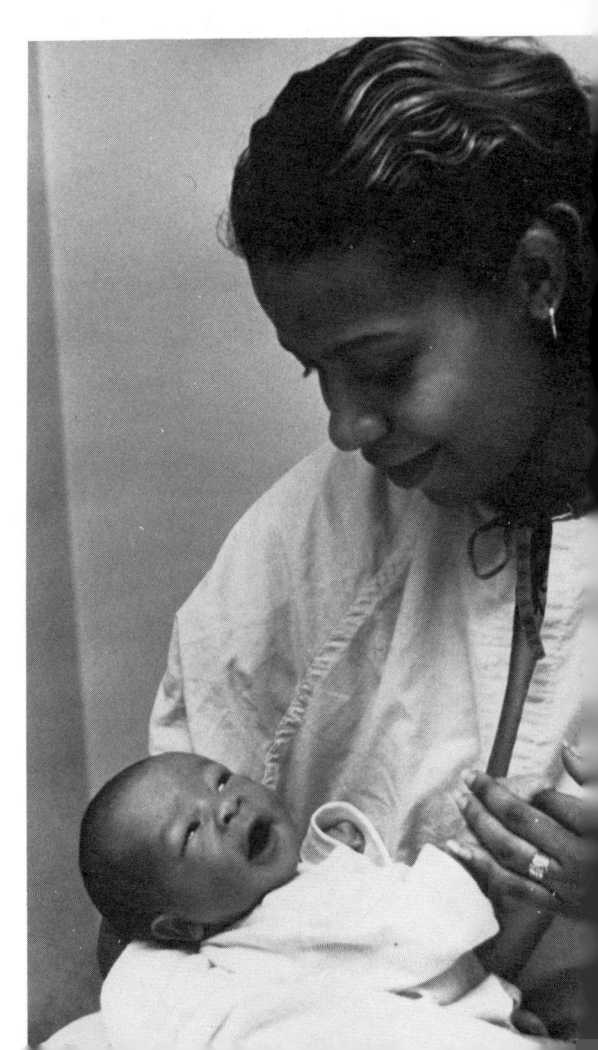

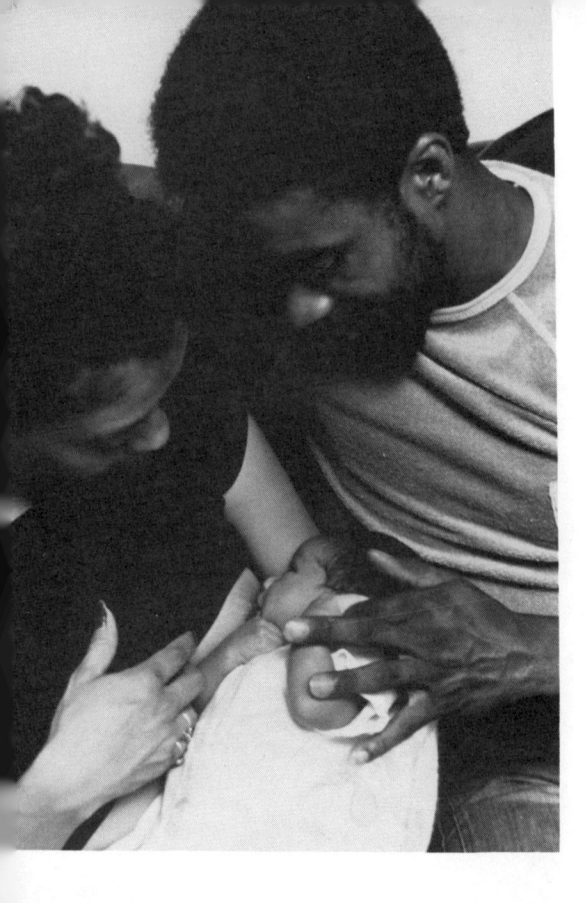

Irritable babies need to be protected from excessive noise and light until their nervous systems become more mature. The environment should be as quiet and simple as possible. Since starts and trembles may work them into an irritable state, they need to be wrapped securely, cuddled, rocked, and soothed with special care.

SOOTHABILITY

One of the most important characteristics of your baby is his ability to be soothed. Babies differ in how easily they are comforted and how much they cry after efforts to calm them have begun. Some babies quiet themselves. Other babies are constantly fussy and spend a great deal of their time crying, even after extensive consoling efforts. These babies are especially hard on first mothers, for the mothers become discouraged and feel badly about their mothering skills. These babies need special support and help.

Don't blame yourself or feel guilty if you have a fussy baby. He is making a lot of physical adjustments during his first weeks of life. Do all you can to comfort him and then accept the situation realistically. Tune in to your instincts when your baby is crying. If you feel strongly that you must pick him up, pick him up. If you feel that you have done everything possible, don't be worried about letting him cry for a few minutes.

Being aware of and responsive to your newborn's messages takes flexibility on your part. In turn, your baby learns to adjust to your behavior. Over the weeks and months, as your baby matures and changes, you will need flexibility and sensitivity to respond to this constantly changing relationship.

When you discover your baby's individual style, find a compromise between your style and his that is mutually satisfactory. Try to avoid being rigid in either your own requirements or your perception of your infant's needs. Do what makes you and your baby feel the best and enjoy each other the most. Success is when both you and your baby enjoy your play periods together. What you do as a parent is not as important to your baby as *how* you do it. The very fact that you care and are concerned about your baby is the most important message you can send.

4.

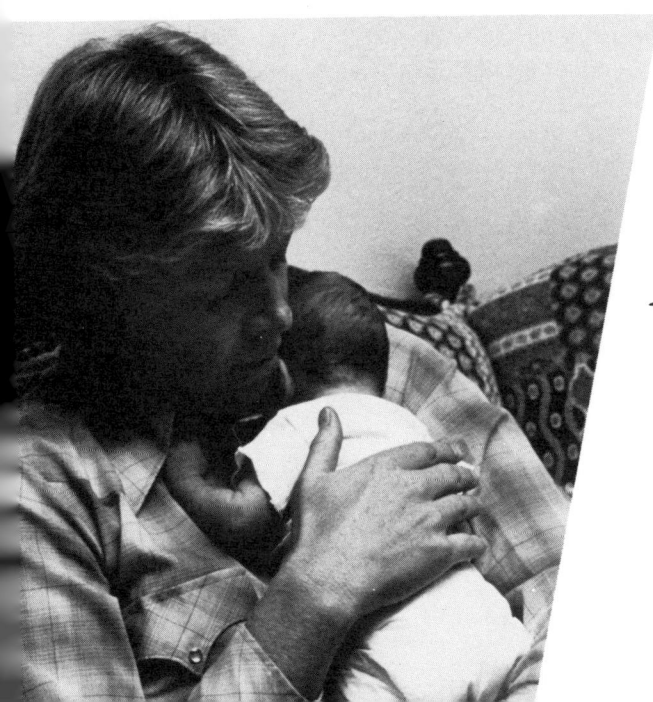

Soothing Your Newborn

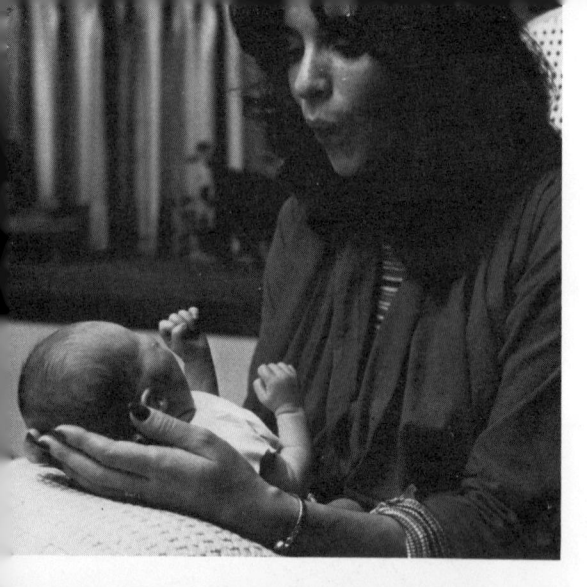

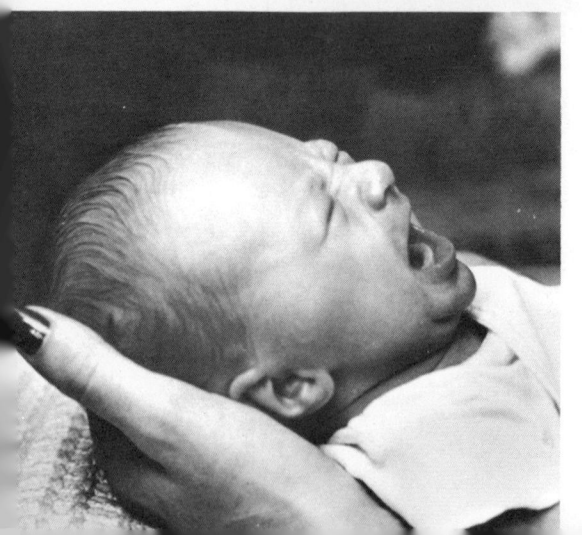

During the first few weeks of life, most of your parenting tasks, other than those of feeding, revolve around comforting and soothing your infant. There are many different ways of consoling babies. In those first few weeks you will begin to learn which ways are most effective in soothing your baby.

WHAT DOES YOUR BABY'S CRY MEAN?

Signal to Express Needs

Your baby's cry is her signal to you that she needs attention. Your quick response will build trust. Crying is a potent stimulus, and there is no other period in your child's life when she is more in control of the attention she receives than during these early weeks. One researcher showed that in four out of five instances, it was the newborn who initiated the action.

Your baby may cry because she is hungry or uncomfortable, or lonely and wanting company, or because she has become overly excited and can't handle the stimulus. She may cry because she is tired but can't get to sleep by herself.

In the beginning when your baby cries your soothing efforts will be based on how long it has been since the last feeding; how adequate that feeding was; and consequently, whether the cry means hunger. However, as time passes, you will begin to hear specific qualities in your baby's cry that will help you differentiate the meanings of particular crying patterns. It will take some time, and may be very frustrating, but you can, through careful observation, begin to understand what she is telling you. Many times even your newborn does not know why she is crying.

HUNGER

When your baby is hungry, her crying signal is usually loud and hard. She will wave her arms and legs vigorously and will root or suck at her fingers, hands, or anything she can get her hands on. When you feed her, the crying stops.

EXHAUSTION

If your baby cries after she has been fed and you have checked her diaper, clothing, et cetera, she may simply be exhausted. Lay her down, let her cry for a while (up to 15 minutes) and see if she can settle herself down. Rocking the crib and patting her back may help.

SICK OR IN PAIN

A baby who is sick may give a high screeching wail or may whimper quietly. If you feel that this crying is "different" from her normal sounds, do not hesitate to call your doctor.

OTHER REASONS

Other times your baby may be in an uncomfortable position, and when she is moved she will stop crying. Her diapers may be wet or irritating and, when they are changed, she stops crying. She may be bored, and when you come over and pay attention to her, she stops crying. Your baby may be overdressed and too hot, or underdressed and cold, and when you take care of this situation, she stops crying. Your baby may simply need cuddling, and when you pick her up and love her, she responds by stopping her crying.

Fussiness

Some babies just seem to have a fussy period at the same time each day. These periods usually occur in the late afternoon or early evening, just when the parents would like a little peace and quiet together. This fussy period usually takes place no matter what you do. It is important to remember that this is a stage that will pass as your baby matures.

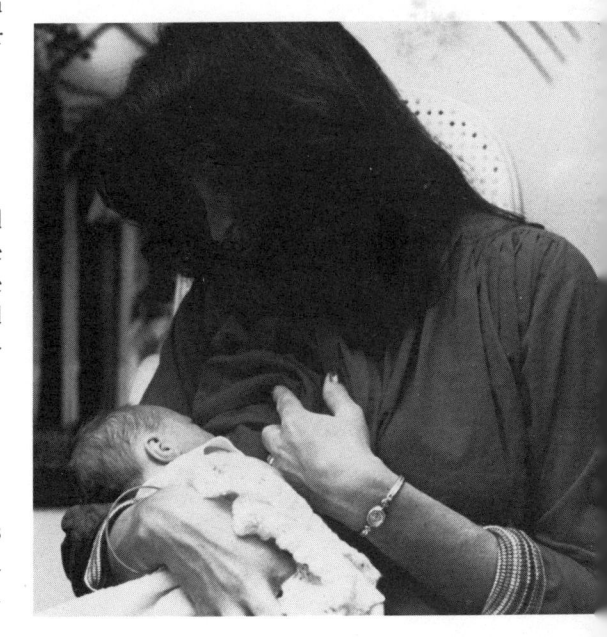

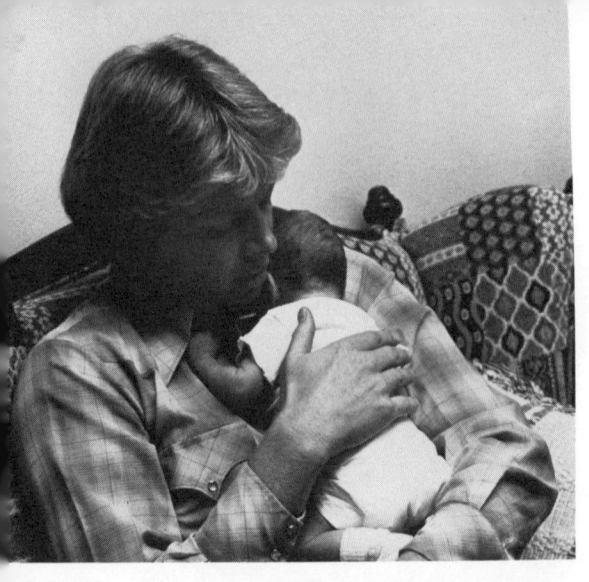

Length and Frequency

Babies differ in how long, how frequently, and how intensely they cry. An irritable baby who cries often and long usually gets more attention from her mother than one who is placid. However, the placid baby who cries very little may be in greater need of stimulation, but receives less because she calls for less.

Intervention

For some babies, early soothing intervention helps to reduce the tension and offer comfort. In general, if your baby is picked up soon after she starts to cry, it takes much less time for her to stop than if she is allowed to work herself into a more frenzied state.

Crying Decreases

As your baby matures, her crying periods decrease, and her alert awake times increase. This results in more time for playing and pleasurable social interaction. In the first three months your baby probably cries a little less than eight minutes each hour. By the end of the first year her crying decreases to a little over four minutes per hour.

SOOTHING YOUR NEWBORN

Your baby's ability to be soothed is as powerful as her cry. Her response is a reward for your efforts. Every baby responds differently to different techniques of consoling. Many newborns can be soothed easily, but others demand vigorous interventions.

Soothing Techniques

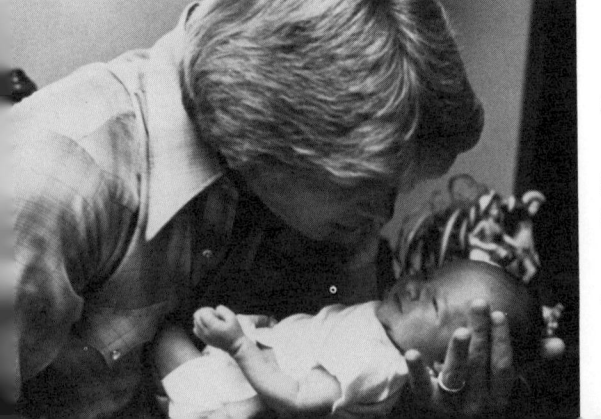

To find out what best suits your baby's need to be comforted, try progressively more active techniques. Holding and consoling works well for some infants, while others need to be left alone to work through their overstimulation.

LEAVE BABY ALONE

Some babies are capable of soothing themselves. They do not need and in fact may be annoyed by vigorous soothing techniques. So, when your baby is crying, first wait 15 seconds to see if she is able to quiet herself. She may do this by putting her hand to her mouth and sucking on her fist or tongue, or she may use a visual or auditory stimulus to focus on. If self-quieting does not occur, be ready to try other techniques to help soothe her.

SHOW FACE

Some babies are consoled when a parent shows his or her face. As your baby is crying, lean over her bassinet or crib, get your face in her line of vision, and see if she will focus on you and calm down.

TALK TO YOUR BABY

Some babies quiet down if they see your face and hear your voice. So, when you get your baby to look at you, try crooning, singing, or talking to her. Ask her what is wrong and what she would like you to do to help her. Keep talking in a soothing, comforting voice.

SWADDLING

Some babies are soothed by the security of having a hand placed firmly on their belly, or having one or both of their arms held firmly to their sides. Some babies will quiet down if a blanket is swaddled tightly around their body.

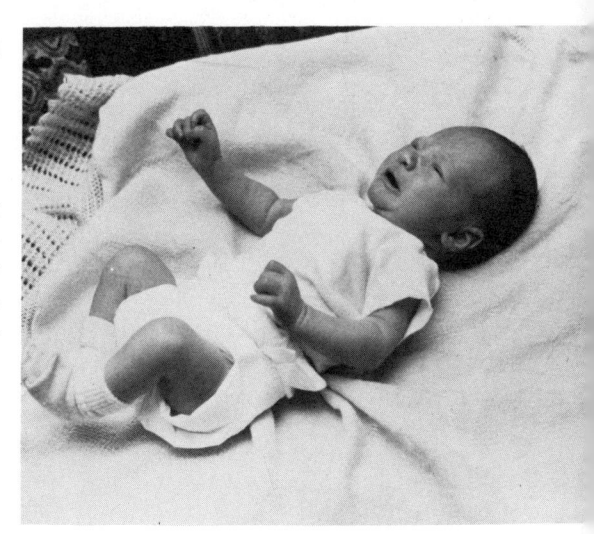

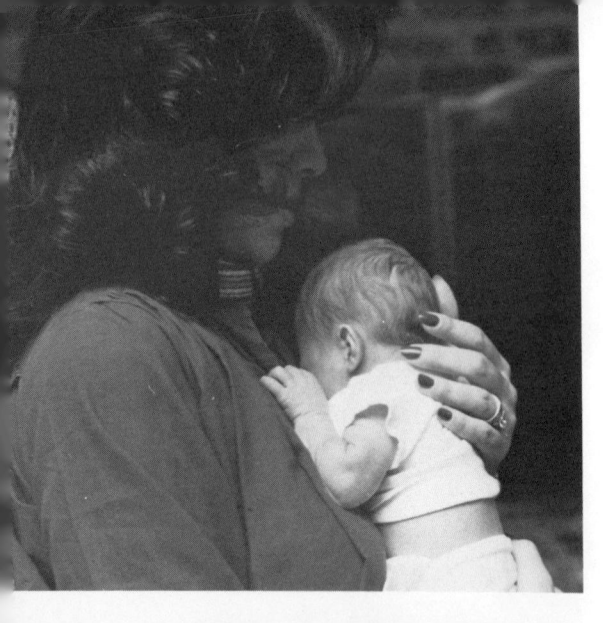

PICK BABY UP

Many babies will quiet down when they are picked up and held. Putting your baby upright against your shoulder close to your body can have a very positive soothing effect. In addition to comforting, this provides your baby with different things to look at. She usually responds with eyes bright, alert, and in focus.

MORE VIGOROUS EFFORTS

Vigorous multiple efforts are needed to soothe some babies. Holding, cuddling, and vigorous rocking, along with tight swaddling, crooning, or even a bottle, breast, or pacifier may be necessary to console the baby. Sometimes such a variety of measures is the only thing that works, and a parent should not feel unhappy or guilty about it. A baby's crying is not the parents' fault; her fussiness and irritability are built in.

OTHER SOOTHING MEASURES

After you have fed, changed, and soothed your baby and she is still crying:

- Check for pins or other physical reasons for discomfort.
- Check for air bubbles.
- Swaddle her in a warm blanket.
- Rub her back and tummy.
- Put her over your shoulder and walk with her.
- Sit in a rocking chair and rock her.
- Croon and talk to her.
- Sing loudly.
- Put her in a sling, backpack, or stroller and go out.
- Make sure she is warm enough.
- Check to see if she is too hot.
- Play with her.

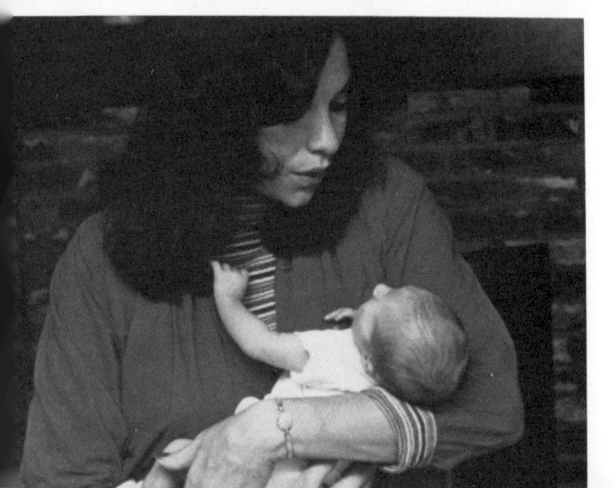

- Put baby in the center of family activities to interest her.
- Give her a warm bath.
- Rock her with a hot water bottle on your lap.
- Put her in a cradle and rock her.
- Give her a pacifier or your finger to suck on.
- Let her alone to sleep.
- Put her in a car and go for a ride.
- Leave her with your husband.
- Go for a walk by yourself.
- Get a baby-sitter and go out with your husband.
- Don't feel guilty.
- Remember, the situation is temporary!

Colic

When your baby has been changed, fed, burped, diapered, bathed, cuddled, walked, and rocked, and you have tried every measure possible to console her without succeeding in stopping her crying, that is colic. With colic, your baby seems to experience attacks of crying about the same time every day; the common time is around 5:00 P.M. Your baby will scream a loud, sustained pitch and does not give up regardless of your soothing efforts. The crying will continue for up to 20 minutes. It may stop and then begin again. Your baby may draw up her knees and elbows in pain. She may pass gas, which will give her some relief. The reasons for colic are vague and varying; there is no one relief measure. Something may work one time for your baby and not another. A mother with a colicky baby must have a variety of measures to try at different times.

FEEDING

Don't let your baby cry excessively before feeding. Burp her before, during, and after her feedings. If you are breast-feeding, do not let the first stream of milk spurt into her mouth, for she will swallow air with it. Release it into a jar and then let her breast-feed. If you are bottle-feeding, check to see that the nipple does not have too big a hole—it may be spurting more milk than she can handle at one time.

TENSION

Colic is catching. You can get it from your baby. The more your baby cries and is inconsolable, the more frustrated, tense, and irritable you become, and the more your baby cries. It is a vicious circle. Try to remain calm, move slowly, speak quietly. When you find yourself becoming uncontrollably tense, leave your baby with your husband, baby-sitter, friend, or neighbor. Take time out with a warm bath, a glass of wine, or a relaxing walk. It is hard, but try to remember that colic is neither your nor your baby's fault and this is only a temporary situation.

5.

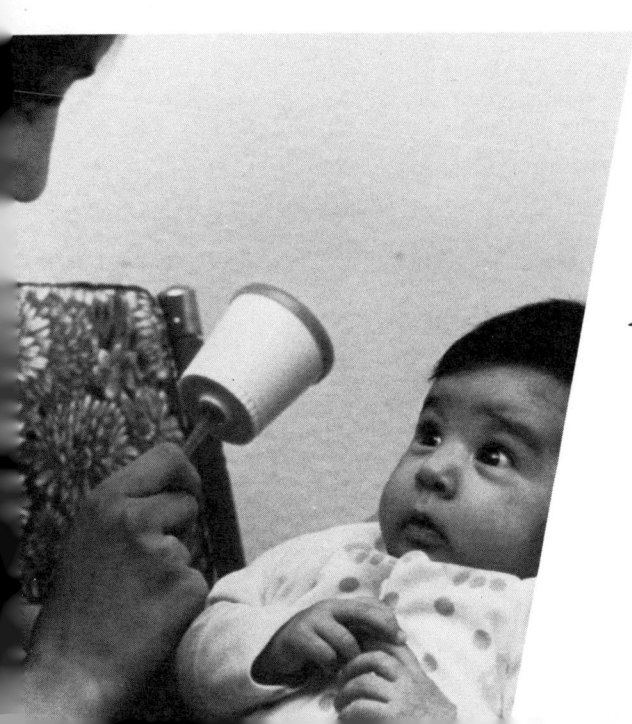

Playing with Your Newborn

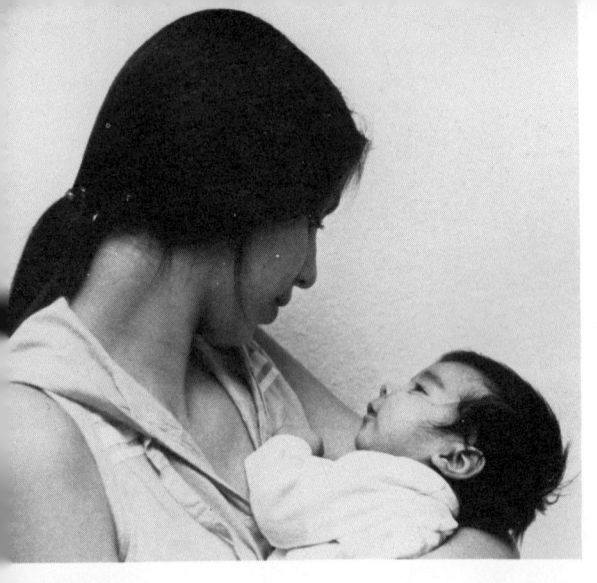

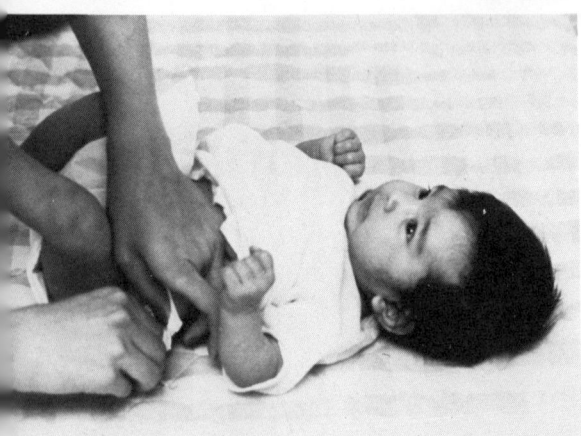

Recent research has shown that your baby is born a social being. When he is only a few minutes old, he already prefers to look at a human face. Only a few hours old, his entire body moves in rhythm to the sound and pattern of a human voice. At the end of a week, your newborn recognizes and prefers your face, voice, touch, and smell over all others. Within a few short weeks, your baby learns how to invite you to play and becomes an expert at maintaining your attention, adjusting the flow of interaction to fit his needs.

Your baby is born with the desire and the capacity to learn. What you do with your face, voice, body, and hands provides your baby with his first experiences in human communication and relationship. Your baby learns through sight, sound, and touch how it feels to be loved, and learns to love in return. He learns by imitating his parents and through his parents' imitating him.

Play between you and your baby is a mutual exchange of joy and fun that builds your baby's knowledge of all things human. As you create new ways to amuse your baby, he learns an increasing variety of responses. The give and take in play provides your baby with the experiences he needs to grow and develop.

PLAYTIME

A play period between infant and parent can last only a few seconds or continue for minutes. Play can take place spontaneously throughout the day, any time your baby's alertness shows he is ready.

Some babies like to play a few minutes before feedings, others during or after feedings. Some babies play best while their parents are diapering or bathing them. Your newborn is alert only about 10 percent of his waking hours during the first weeks of life, although this period more than triples by his third month. When he looks at you or makes a gesture (or later on, when he smiles), he is signaling you that he is ready for play. You can also begin the interaction with a smile or a touch.

THE RHYTHM OF PLAY

There is a synchronization between you and your baby. As you talk, your baby listens; as you touch, he responds; as you look at him, your baby returns a loving gaze. Your baby's body movements are his means of communication. Learning his rhythms is like learning to dance with a new partner; it takes a little time. Parents who are sensitive to these unique rhythms are better able to enjoy parenting.

As you and your baby respond to each other rhythmically, it is much like playing a game in which each takes turns. You may initiate play with a touch or eye contact, and then your baby responds. As you wait for him to respond, watch his face, toes, hands—the rhythm of his body. Either one of you can continue the game with another signal. When your baby has received enough stimulation, he will withdraw, perhaps by yawning or turning away. It is important that you understand that this is also part of the game.

Attention/Nonattention

During his alert active period your baby takes in information from everything in his new environment. With rapt attention, he turns to the stimuli, becomes attentive, focuses, and then loses interest and turns aside. During this "nonattention" time he reviews, organizes, and puts away information for future use. Your baby behaves differently in response to each type of stimulus. Objects present a limited amount of information, while humans offer richness and complexity.

OBJECT

When interacting with an object, your baby beams and reaches his feet and arms toward it. He watches with rapt, fixed, bright expressions on his face. When he has taken in all the information he can handle, he breaks off his attention and turns his eyes and even head and body for a brief period before he comes back for further learning.

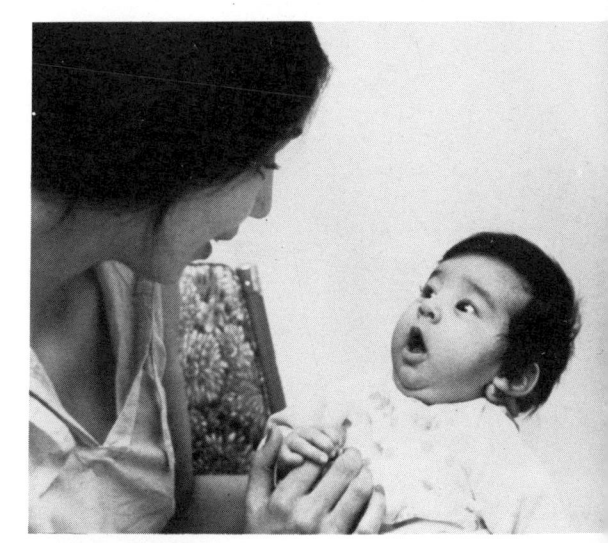

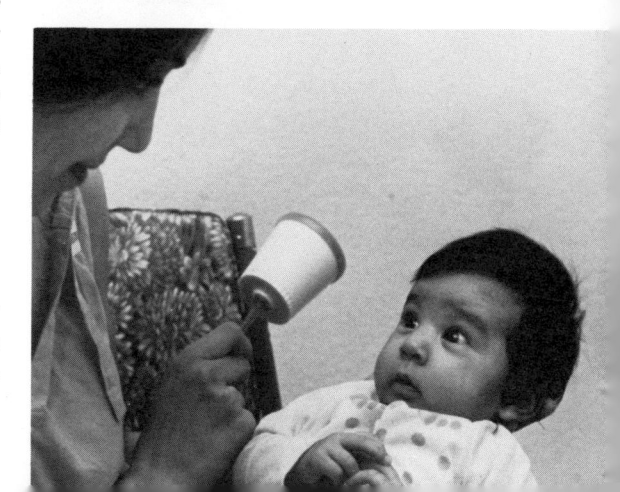

PARENT

When your baby is interacting with you, all parts of his body move in patterns toward and away from you. His eyes focus and his face is bright with interest. When he reaches his limit, instead of abruptly losing interest, he lets his eyes slowly shift from your face and begins a cycle of nonattention in which he seems to recover or readjust. Although he does not look directly at you, all of your movements are in his field of vision. When he is sufficiently recovered and readjusted, he slowly returns his gaze to you and begins a new attention cycle.

LIMITS

These short cycles of attention and nonattention are important parts of the communication between you and your newborn. He will signal a halt when he has become overstimulated and can take no more. Your baby's signals for play and for the amount of stimulus he can handle are the cues that you use to shape your behavior with him. When parents are insensitive to their baby's individual cycle, the infant withdraws his attention and spends most of his time turned away. By not responding to his attention-and-withdrawal pattern and continuing with a steady bombardment of stimuli, you may reinforce withdrawal and decrease the time he pays attention to you.

If the delicate balance of signals and responses is upset, the result can be short and unsatisfying interactions between you and your baby. When your baby seems out of phase with your attempts at interaction, wait for him to come back to a state of attention before continuing the game.

If parents have fixed expectations about their baby's responses, they are sure to meet with frustration. It is important to put aside rigid ideas of "good parenting." Too much stimulation may keep an excitable baby from achieving stability. Too little, from parents who fear spoiling their baby, may fail to meet the baby's needs.

SENSORY EXPERIENCES

Seeing

One of the ways your baby learns about his environment is by looking around. Interesting visual experiences help him learn about and enjoy life and keep him alert and interested. Bring objects close enough for him to see clearly. Provide him with mobiles and crib toys, and use brightly colored posters and wall paper. Carry him to objects that are out of his focus, such as interesting wallpaper or flowers in the garden. Tell him what he is looking at, talk to him about it, and show pleasure to increase his visual alertness and decrease his tendency to be bored. Change your baby's position in bed often so he can see around him, and place him in the middle of family activities.

Although bright, colorful objects and soft, soothing sounds interest your baby, you, the parent, are his best toy. When held in your arms for feeding, he is at the perfect distance to focus on your face, study your outlines, enjoy the contrasts between your eyes and hair and the movement of your lips, mouth, and eyes. He can listen to the changes in your voice, feel your body, and touch your skin and clothing.

Hearing

Hearing is another way your baby receives information about his environment. During his alert period, talk to him. Parents naturally speak more slowly, and use exaggerated tones and emphases to get a baby's attention. He enjoys rattles and bells that make different noises, and the rhythm and soothing qualities of music. It is never too early to start to read to your infant. He finds pleasure in the sounds and rhythms of language and loves to listen while being held and cuddled.

Touching

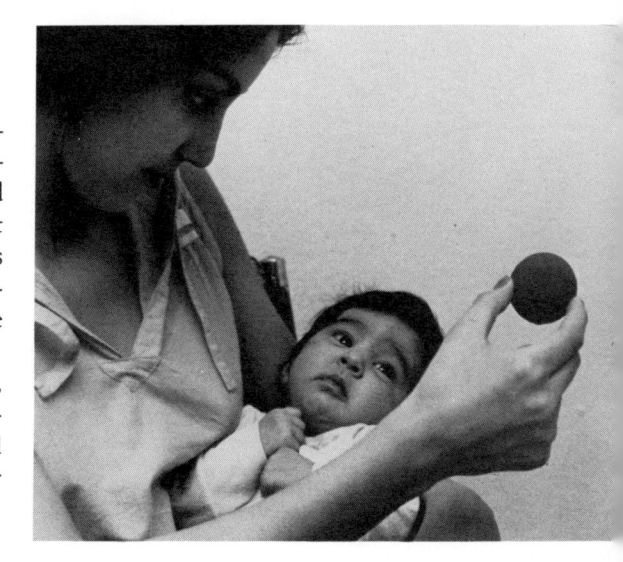

Touch is the best language you can use with your newborn. It conveys better than words your love, warmth, and support. Consider your hands and your body as a means of talking with your baby. From birth, hold your baby close to your skin. Explore his body; touch, fondle, and caress him. Before bathing your baby, massage every part and fold of his body, with or without baby oil. Start from his chest and work over his body, back, buttocks, arms, and legs with soothing, strong, gentle, and firm stroking movements.

During playtime, grasp your baby's hand and pull him toward you gently. He also enjoys having his legs and arms gently stretched. Provide soft cuddly toys for him to hold.

Movement

Your baby derives great pleasure from various kinds of movement. Be sure to rock and bounce him often. Hold him in your arms when you walk or dance, and take him on rides in the stroller or car.

Smelling

Smells fascinate babies, and they encounter new and different ones everywhere they go: food smells, house smells, the outdoors. Two smells a baby can derive great comfort from are the scents of his mother's and father's bodies.

Your baby will grow mentally and emotionally during the first two months as much as he will grow physically. The newborn who is totally occupied with taking in his first sounds, sights, and perceptions will develop in the next two months into a social person who is capable of both taking and giving and who will give you endless hours of delight.

6.

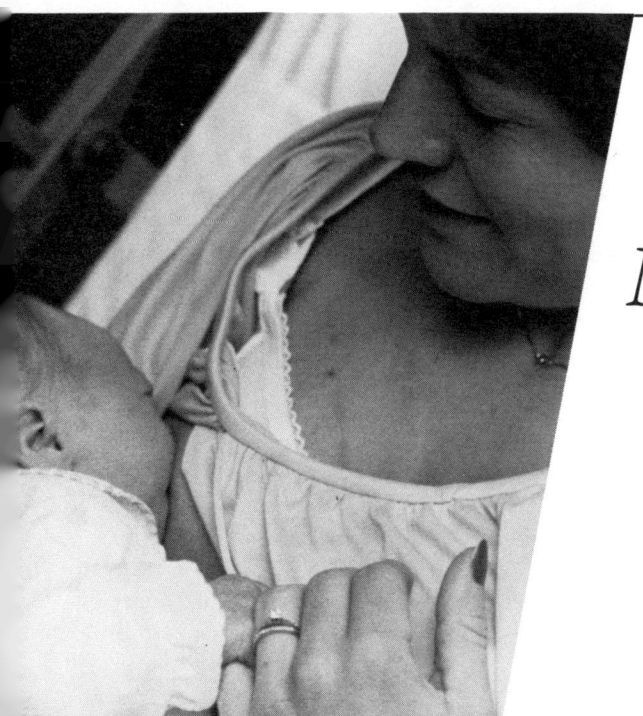

Feeding Your Newborn

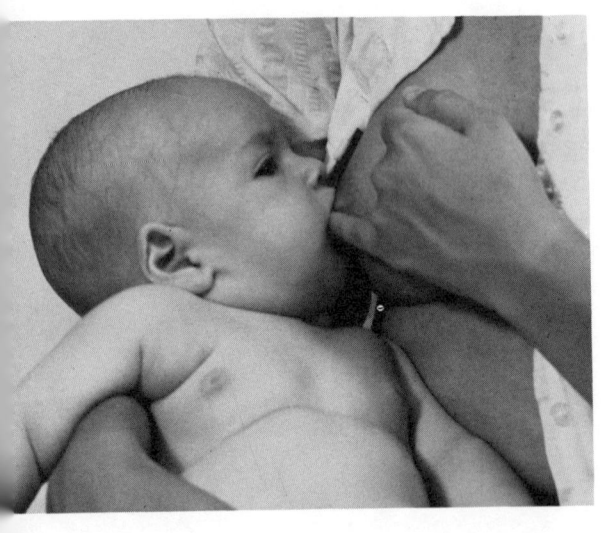

Your baby's most crucial need is for nourishment, whether it is from the breast or the bottle. In your uterus your baby received perfect nourishment in a constant supply. She has never experienced hunger and has never experienced schedules, so she has some adjustments to make.

Whether you breast-feed or bottle-feed, at feeding time you fulfill her needs not only for nourishment but also for sucking, warmth, cuddling, and closeness to you. Approach feeding in a calm, relaxed, and unhurried mood. Take special care to find a comfortable position, and take advantage of this time to treat yourself to a glass of juice, milk, or tea.

For the first few weeks it is best to feed your baby whenever she tells you she needs it. You may have from one to four hours between feedings. By the end of the first month, most babies have established a definite schedule and want from six to ten feedings a day. As you can see, you spend a great deal of time feeding your baby during the first few months of her life.

BREAST-FEEDING

Breast-feeding may not be for every woman. But for those who do wish to breast-feed, full support, encouragement, and assistance should be available. Emotional support from the father is an important component of successful breast-feeding. The birth of a child can be emotionally upsetting to a man. He may experience overwhelming feelings of responsibility and isolation. It is important for a couple to share their concerns and search together for information, skills, and support.

A supportive obstetrician is essential to a woman who wishes to breast-feed. Many women also find support in groups, such as La Leche League, whose members have successfully breast-fed their babies and who share their experiences with new mothers.

Breast-feeding has several advantages for the baby:

1. Human milk is best suited to the digestive system of the human baby. It has highly digestible protein, fat, vitamins, and minerals.
2. Breast-fed babies are less susceptible to respiratory infections, diarrhea, and allergies and, in later life, may experience a lower incidence of obesity, cardiovascular

disease, gastroenteritis, and dental problems.
3. Mother's milk provides a baby with a period of resistance to viral and bacterial infections.
4. The cuddling and fondling that naturally accompany breast-feeding give the baby emotional benefits that help to build her security, emotional stability, and the ability to give and receive love in later life.

Advantages for the mother are:

1. Less physical effort once breast-feeding has been established: no formulas, bottles, nipples, sterilizing, mixing, or heating. Breast milk naturally contains the correct ingredients at the right temperature.
2. Human milk is more economical than prepared formula.
3. Night feedings are more convenient for everyone.
4. Nursing helps your uterus return to normal more rapidly.

Physiology

Your breast is a large gland capable of converting the nutrients from your blood into milk. The size of your breast is determined by the amount of fat and has nothing to do with your ability to breast-feed. Milk is produced in glands called the alveoli, which are located deep in the fatty parts of your breast. These glands increase in size during pregnancy, when large amounts of the hormones estrogen and progesterone are present in your bloodstream. After your baby's birth, the decrease of these hormones signals the milk glands to begin their function.

Milk Production

When your baby sucks at your nipple, its sensitive nerve endings send the message through your nervous system to your brain, where your pituitary gland is stimulated. The pituitary gland then releases the hormone prolactin into your bloodstream to stimulate

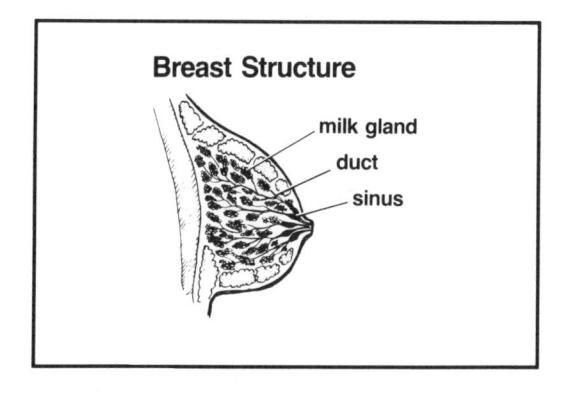

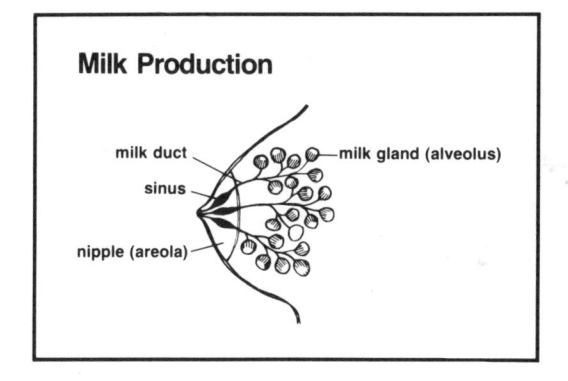

Breast Structure

- milk gland
- duct
- sinus

Milk Production

- milk duct
- sinus
- nipple (areola)
- milk gland (alveolus)

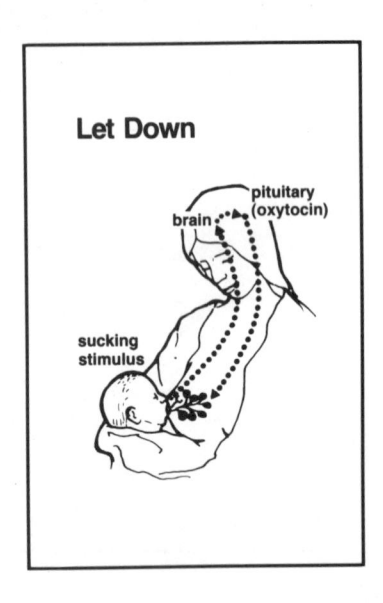

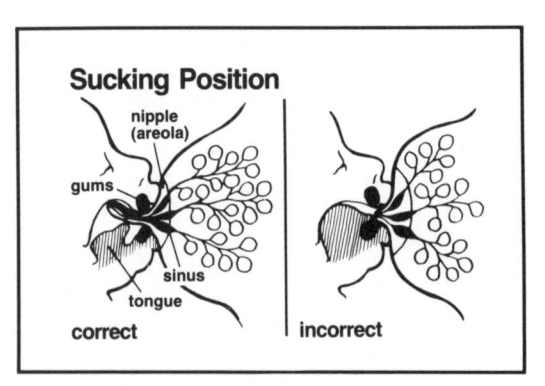

your milk glands. Bandlike contracting cells around each milk gland squeeze milk out through the ducts and into the milk sinuses. This is called the "let-down" reflex. Shortly after your baby begins to nurse, the sucking sends another message through your nervous system to your brain, which stimulates the release of another hormone, oxytocin, into your bloodstream. When oxytocin reaches the milk glands, it activates the contracting cells to squeeze the milk out through the ducts to the milk sinuses under the areola or nipple, where it is easily available to your baby. Even though your milk glands are capable of producing large amounts of milk, without the let-down reaction, your baby would not get sufficient milk to nourish him.

Since the let down is an integral part of your nervous system's functioning, any negative emotion, such as tension, fear, embarrassment, anxiety, or anger, causes your pituitary gland to secrete adrenalin, which can inhibit oxytocin, thus off-setting let down. A relaxed and rested mother helps the let down function effectively.

Milk Supply

The amount of milk you can produce is determined primarily by how much is sucked or emptied out. The more your breasts are emptied, the more milk they produce. Frequent and extensive nursing produces a maximum supply of milk. On the other hand, brief, infrequent feedings result in a minimum supply.

Frequent and extensive nursing ensures that the milk is drained from the ducts and sinuses, so that little excess remains. Inadequate drainage of the milk ducts may cause engorgement and even infection. Short, infrequent feedings, giving supplemental food, milk, or water, or even fatigue can cause such problems.

Correct Nursing

Successful breast-feeding depends not only on you, the mother, but on a cooperating infant as well. A baby who is nursing correctly grasps the dark area, or areola, which covers the milk sinuses, sucks your nipple into her mouth, gently compresses her gums around the milk sinuses, and squeezes the milk into her mouth. Slow, rhythmic, satisfied sounds come from her.

A baby who is nursing incorrectly grasps only the end of your nipple. The milk sinuses do not reach into her mouth and she cannot get the milk out. Your nipple becomes sore and your baby is left hungry and frustrated.

First Nursing

Many babies have little energy for eating and digesting as they recover from labor and delivery. Whether your baby wants to nurse immediately or not, early contact between the two of you helps to ensure a more successful breast-feeding experience. Rooming-in, where the baby remains in the hospital room with the mother, is especially helpful in making a good start in breast-feeding.

You may choose to nurse your baby in either a sitting or lying position. If you are sitting, place a pillow in your lap to bring your baby up to the level of your nipple. If you feed lying down, lay your baby at the level of your nipple. Gently bring your baby to your breast. Grasp your areola between your thumb and forefinger and gently stroke back and forth on your baby's cheek with the nipple. She will turn to grasp it. Even though your baby may not begin nursing immediately, her licking of your nipple causes a release of prolactin and oxytocin into your bloodstream. This also signals your uterus to contract, thus reducing postpartum bleeding.

Nurse your baby frequently for short periods in the beginning to allow your nipples to toughen—approximately five minutes at each breast the first day; five to ten minutes the second day; and ten to fifteen minutes the third. It's important to nurse long enough from the very beginning to establish the let-down reflex. Your baby should nurse from both breasts at each feeding to ensure adequate drainage.

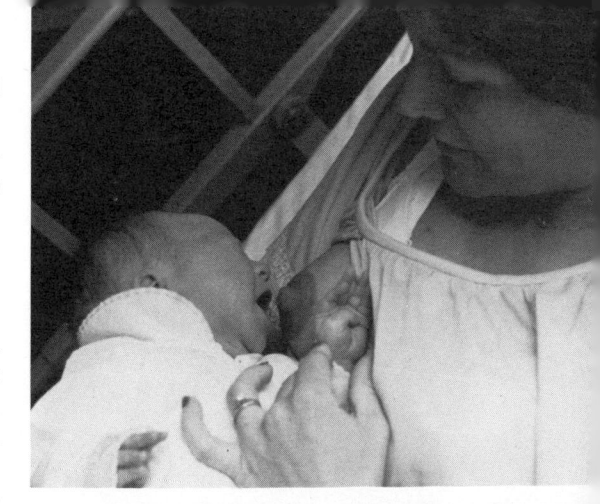

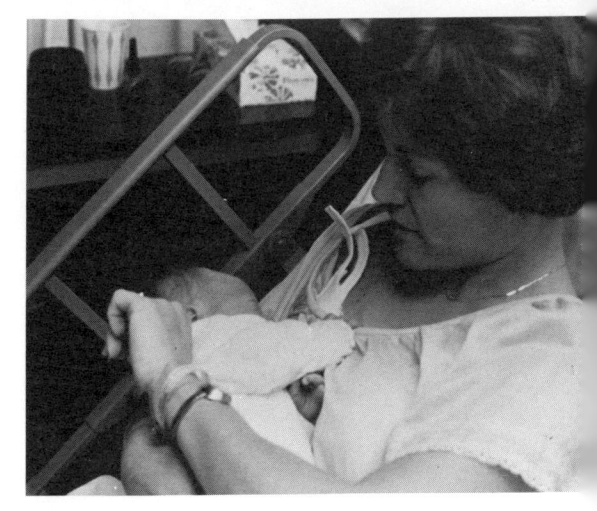

To break suction painlessly, gently place your little finger in the corner of your baby's mouth between your nipple and her lips and press against your breast. Bubble your baby before putting her on your other breast. Hold her in a sitting position and gently pat her back. When nursing on your side, you can produce the same effect by placing your baby on your chest and rubbing her back.

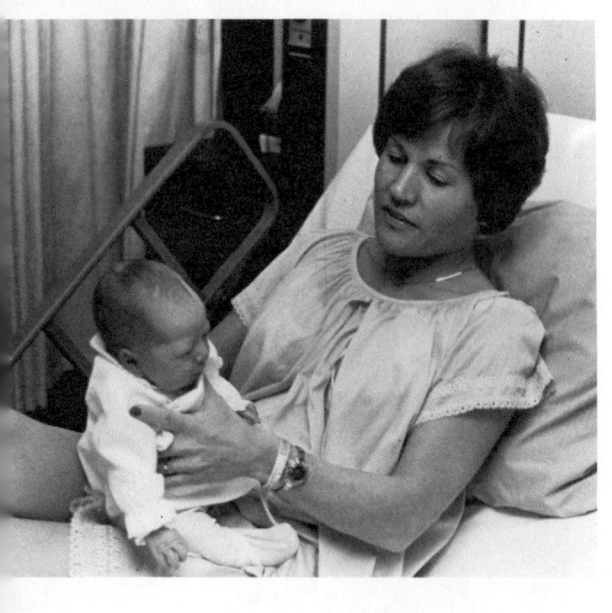

To ensure complete drainage and an adequate milk supply, always begin your next feeding on the breast that was nursed last. The night feeding is always important in ensuring complete drainage and establishing a good milk supply.

When your nipples become accustomed to nursing, you can allow your baby to nurse fifteen minutes or longer on each breast.

Make sure you drink the fluids you need for successful breast-feeding.

You can usually be confident your baby is getting enough milk if she has six to eight good, wet diapers a day after the first day or so, and if she seems contented. Normal bowel movements are runny, light in color and milk-smelling, with frequency anywhere from several times a day to several times a week.

Remember, it takes time to establish breast-feeding. Both you and your baby are participants in a learning process. Many times new babies are not very hungry during their first few days. Take your time, relax, and enjoy it.

Problems: Baby

You're sure to encounter some moments of frustration when breast-feeding your new baby. Some common problems are:

CRYING

A crying baby cannot breast-feed. Try to calm her down by rubbing her back, rocking or cuddling her, walking or singing while holding her. Taking a bath with the baby might also help.

SLEEPINESS

A sleepy baby cannot suck properly to get sufficient milk at a feeding. To wake a baby, uncover her and expose her tummy to air. If this doesn't work, try rubbing her feet, patting her hands, or rubbing her head.

VIGOROUS NURSING

A baby who nurses too vigorously may swallow air, causing gas and colic. To slow nursing, burp your baby before you start, and again when changing breasts. You can nurse for shorter, more frequent periods or use only one breast at each feeding. Stop nursing for a few seconds at the time of the most intense let down.

WEAK NURSING

A weak nurser (such as a premature baby) may become exhausted and discouraged. Nurse the weak nurser more frequently. Hand-express milk into her mouth to get your breast soft and to help initiate nursing. Be sure to give lots of body contact to stimulate her.

COLIC

Check the baby for comfort; you may be overfeeding her. Nurse her for shorter, more frequent periods. Rock, cuddle, and soothe her.

SICKNESS

Call your doctor if you suspect she is sick, but keep nursing. Your breast milk is the best nourishment if your baby is sick.

Problems: Mother

You may also face some problems while trying to breast-feed. It is very important that your doctor supports breast-feeding and is familiar with the complications that might occur.

LET DOWN

Rest and relaxation are imperative for let down to take place. If you are having difficulty with let down, massage your breasts; take a hot bath or use a hot water bottle; or take a glass of juice, wine, or beer to relax you. Use your childbirth techniques of slow breathing and relaxation.

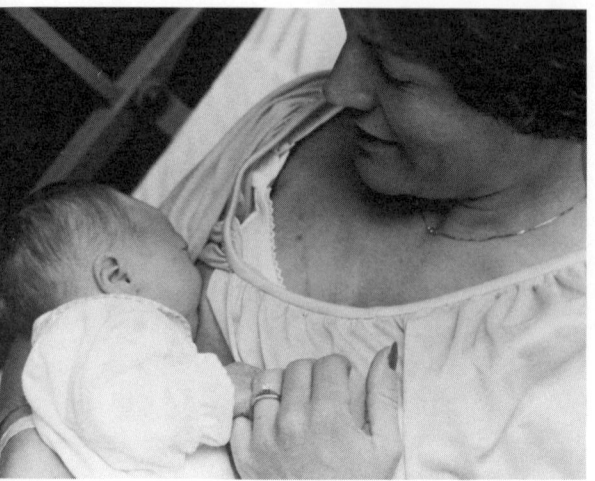

MILK SUPPLY

Frequent, prolonged nursing, lots of liquids, and a good diet will help to ensure a good supply of milk. To build up your milk supply, increase your fluid intake and increase the frequency of nursing.

ENGORGEMENT

A vigorously nursing baby can often overstimulate your milk supply during the first few weeks. Nursing soon after birth and frequently can help prevent engorgement. If engorgement does take place, continue breast-feeding and contact your doctor. Try ice bags to decrease swelling between feedings and apply warmth to your breast before feedings to enhance let down. One of the best ways to do this is to make your own heat vacuum pump. Take a wide-mouth glass jar that has been washed and heated with hot water. Pour off the hot water and place the mouth of the jar over your areola. As the jar cools, excess milk is drawn off. Throw away this milk. Try this after and before nursings or whenever you need relief.

INFECTION

The possibility of infection, or mastitis, can be minimized by good drainage, frequent nursing, prevention of cracked nipples and lots of rest. If infection does occur, call your doctor immediately, but continue breast-feeding. Take prescribed medicine and nurse using your infected breast first and frequently. Apply heat, using baths or a hot water bottle, and go to bed.

SORE NIPPLES

For sore nipples, offer your baby short, more frequent nursings, since less vigorous nursing will occur if your baby is not so hungry. Expose your nipples to the air and use a light application of hydrous lanolin ointment on them. Crushed ice in a washcloth can provide relief.

Nursing After a Cesarean

If you had a cesarean childbirth, you can still breast-feed your baby, even though getting started may take a little more time and patience. The aftereffects of the anesthesia will slow you down somewhat, and you will need assistance in caring for your baby—with lifting, changing from one breast to the other, and changing positions. Your husband can be a great help at this time. Make sure you drink the fluids you need for successful breast-feeding. Having a cesarean does not change the fact that your breasts will begin their process of producing milk once the placenta is gone from the uterus and the pregnancy hormones decrease.

One of the most important factors in breast-feeding after a cesarean is finding a comfortable position. Once you are comfortable, have your baby brought to you. Supporting her head with your arms, bring her up to your breast. You may use a pillow under her body to keep her off your stitches and, at the same time, give her easiest access to your breast. The effect of breast-feeding on your uterus, stimulating it to contract and revert to its normal size, is significant to your recovery from a cesarean delivery.

Nutrition

Though milk can be made in the absence of good nutrition, its quality eventually becomes poor. Only you can provide the nutrients your baby needs to thrive and grow. Make sure you give your body the proteins, carbohydrates, fats, vitamins, and minerals so necessary for growth and development by eating the following foods daily:

- MILK: 1 to 1½ quarts (4 to 6 cups) of Vitamin-D fortified milk. One cup of yogurt, buttermilk, custard, or pudding equals 1 cup of whole milk. Cottage cheese (1⅓ cups equals 1 cup milk) or hard cheese such as cheddar (1½ ounces equals 1 cup milk) make good substitutes.
- MEAT: Four servings (8 ounces) of lean cooked meat, fish, or poultry. One 2-ounce serving of meat is equivalent to 2 eggs, ½ cup of cottage cheese, 2 slices of cheese, 4 tablespoons of peanut butter, or ¾ cup dried beans, peas, or lentils.
- VEGETABLES: Two 6-ounce servings of green or dark green leafy vegetables.
- CEREALS: Four servings. One slice of whole-grain or enriched bread is equal to ½ cup pasta, grits, or brown rice. One muffin, dumpling, pancake or waffle, 2 corn tortillas, or a 2-inch square of cornbread are all equivalent to 1 slice of bread.
- VITAMIN C: One serving (6 ounces) high in Vitamin C such as citrus fruits, berries, melons, green peppers, tomatoes, or cabbage.
- OTHER: At least one additional serving of any fruit, vegetable, or potato.

Breast-feeding Hints

- Most babies need help in learning how to start breast-feeding.
- Always begin each breast-feeding session with the breast last used.
- Use both breasts at each feeding.
- It is common for a newborn to go to sleep during feeding. Wake her up.
- You may experience uterine cramping during breast-feeding.
- It takes time for both mother and baby to establish a successful routine.

- Breast milk looks thin, bluish, and watery because it does not have a large fat content.
- Breast-fed babies need more frequent feeding than bottle-fed babies.
- Your breast size returns to normal after breast-feeding is established.
- Your baby will go through growth spurts and need more milk.
- Your breasts' milk production will take several days to catch up with your baby's increased needs.
- Frequent feedings help establish a better supply of milk.
- Plenty of rest and relaxation is vital to breast-feeding.
- Drink twice as many fluids as you normally do.
- Loose, yellow, cheeselike stools are normal for the breast-fed baby.
- If your breasts leak, press the palm of your hand against them to stop the flow.
- Do not take any medication, unless prescribed by your doctor.
- Do not take birth control pills while breast-feeding.
- Breast-fed babies do not need solid foods until six months old.

BOTTLE-FEEDING

Although breast milk has many advantages, many mothers prefer to bottle-feed their babies and have sound reasons for doing so. Whether you breast-feed or bottle-feed, the most important ingredient of the feeding experience is the holding, warmth, cuddling, skin-to-skin contact, and face-to-face position your baby experiences.

Those who choose bottle-feeding do so because:

1. It is easier to establish bottle-feeding than breast-feeding.
2. Other people can feed the baby.
3. The father can give night feedings.
4. Some mothers do not wish to breast-feed.
5. Some mothers do not have the information and support they need to enjoy breast-feeding.

Formulas

There are many types of formulas: canned cow's milk, Similac, powdered formula, liquid formula, soy formula. However, a formula suitable for one baby may cause gas, spitting up, vomiting, constipation, diarrhea, or allergy in another. Your doctor, nurse, or clinic will advise you concerning the type of formula to feed your baby. Whatever formula you choose, it is essential that you follow their specific directions to ensure your baby a well-balanced diet.

Equipment

There is no one right style of bottle, but the style of nipple is important. Try to find one that is designed to resemble the human nipple. It is healthier for your baby's mouth, for it makes her work harder to get her milk, unlike the common straight nipple that shoots milk into her mouth.

The size of the hole in the nipple is crucial. If the hole is too large, the baby will suck the milk faster than she can swallow it. As she gulps in the milk, air will also be gulped in, causing gas and colic. Further, when the milk flow is too fast, it does not allow her to develop her mouth and jaw muscles by sucking. If the nipple hole is too small, your baby will become exhausted and discouraged and not get enough milk. You can adjust milk flow by buying nipples without holes and starting with a small hole, enlarging it if the flow is too slow and your baby is working too hard or is not getting enough to satisfy her.

Wash the equipment with soap or detergent, and rinse and dry it well. Be sure that all old formula is removed with a brush, especially inside the bottles and nipple holes. Running the equipment through the dishwasher will sterilize it.

Preparation

Make only one day's supply of formula at a time and throw away any that is left over. The bacteria growth in milk can cause your baby an intestinal upset. For the first six weeks boil all the water for two minutes, then cool it. Pour the required amount of cool water into a clean container. Measure the portion of formula and mix. Remember, to ensure your baby's balanced diet of nutrients, vitamins, and minerals, dilute formula only as directed: measure liquids carefully and use level measurements of powdered ingredients. Do not change proportions of ingredients for any reason without contacting your doctor or clinic, or your baby may have serious intestinal problems as a result.

TEMPERATURE

For a newborn baby, warm the formula to room temperature. You can either heat the bottle in a saucepan of water or run warm water over the bottle. Remember not to leave the milk out to warm up, since it is the perfect medium for bacterial growth. When your baby gets older, you can give her formula right from the refrigerator if she will take it. When you are going out, you can keep the bottle cold by wrapping it in layers of paper. If you are going to be out more than two hours, take along cans of ready-to-feed formula, which you can open right before feeding.

Always remember, with each feeding, one of the things you are giving your baby is love. *Never* prop a bottle in her mouth—always give it to her in your arms with the warmth, cuddling, and attention that only you can give. If you leave a bottle left propped in a baby's mouth over a period of time, you can cause later tooth decay.

Bottle-feeding Hints

- Be sure your baby feels your warm skin and cuddling while you feed her.
- Hold the bottle so that most of the nipple is in your baby's mouth at an angle so that the milk fills the nipple and your baby does not swallow air.
- If your baby falls asleep while you are feeding her, wake her up.
- Burp your baby halfway through each feeding and after each feeding.
- Break suction when you pull the nipple from your baby's mouth by inserting your finger between her mouth and the nipple.

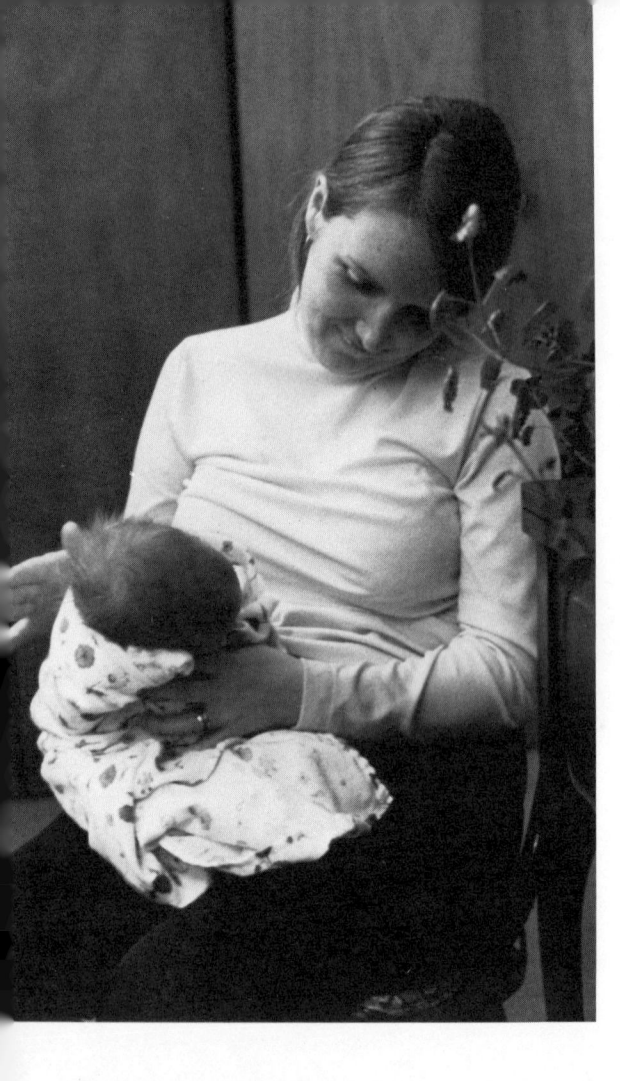

- Don't rush the feeding; be gentle, patient, and take your time.
- Your baby is getting enough when you get six or more wet diapers a day.
- Your baby's stools will vary with the formula.
- Do not rush solid foods.
- Don't overfeed your baby.

Burping/Bubbling

To help your baby get rid of any excess air in her system, burp or bubble her after each feeding. The traditional way is to hold her up with her tummy near your shoulder and gently pat her on her back. You can also burp or bubble your baby in a sitting position, with one hand firmly on her stomach and the other patting her back. A little spitting up is perfectly normal. It usually occurs after a feeding and is caused by an air bubble. If your baby spits up a great deal, she may be overeating. Sometimes it helps if you burp her before feeding, during the feeding, and after the feeding as well.

7.

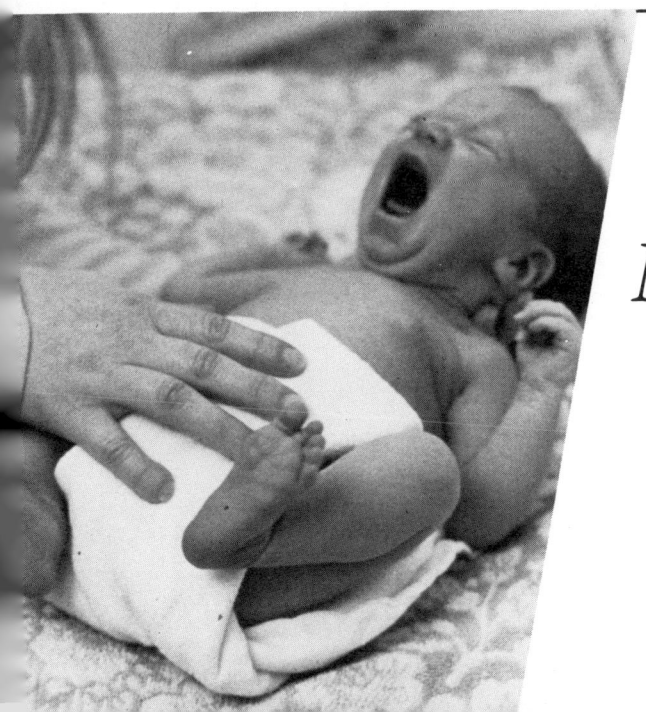

Caring for Your Newborn

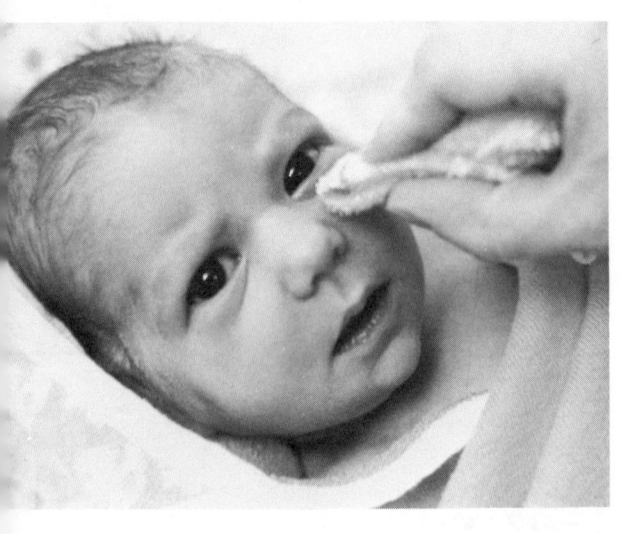

CLEANING

The First Bath

Bathing during the first week consists only of sponging your baby with a mild soap or just water. He should not be placed in a tub of water until his umbilical cord has dropped off and the stump is completely healed. This usually takes from seven to nine days.

First, gather all the materials you'll need: a mild soap, baby shampoo, a washcloth or sponge, a towel, a diaper, pins, cotton swabs, ointment (Desitin or lanolin), and a basin of warm water. The room should be warm—72–80 °F.—and free from drafts. The bath water should be about 98 °F., or comfortably warm when you put your elbow in the water.

Lay your baby on a padded counter and, to avoid upsetting him, keep his body covered for warmth. Never, never leave him alone even for a moment: even the smallest of babies can work their way off unguarded surfaces. Your baby will probably learn to roll over long before you expect it.

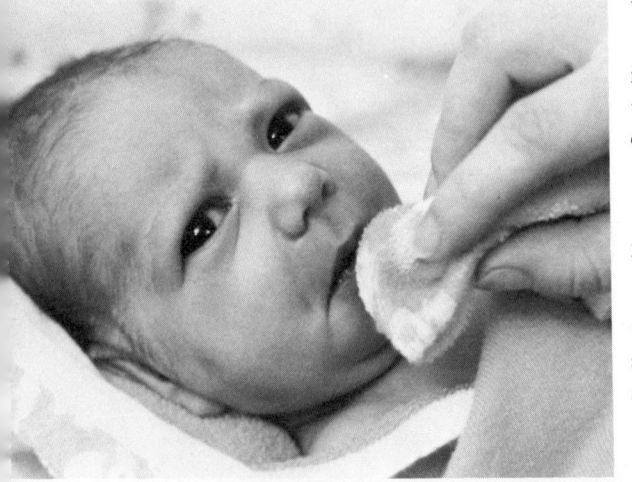

EYES

Wash his eyes first with a clean cloth, starting at the inner part of the eye and sponging toward his ear. There may be swelling from the birth, but it usually disappears within two or three days. A nonirritating antibiotic applied to your baby's eyes after birth may cause whitish matter to appear in their corners.

MOUTH

Wash the outer surfaces of the mouth with a cloth. It is not necessary to clean inside the mouth. You may see some raised white plaque on the roof of your baby's mouth and also note that the outer lining of his lips peels during the first weeks. But conditions are normal.

EARS AND NOSE

Gently wash the outside of his ears and nose. You may use a cotton swab on the outside, but *never* go into the inner areas.

FACE

To wash his face, use a moist washcloth, but no soap, since your baby's facial skin is extremely delicate. Support his head with one hand, and with the other use a firm but gentle stroke. Do not cover his face or you will frighten him. Wash his forehead, nose, cheeks, and around his mouth and chin.

HAIR

Use soapy hands to wash his head, using a gentle rotary motion. Many mothers are concerned about damaging the soft spot, or fontanel. Don't worry; it is protected by tough membranes. Pour water over the scalp and be sure to rinse all the soap out thoroughly. Brush his scalp with a soft baby brush. Avoid using oil. Cradle cap, or dry, flaky scalp, occurs often and is not a sign of a negligent mother.

BODY

After finishing the head and face, gently wash his body with a mild soap, paying special attention to the folds under his arms and in the groin.

BUTTOCKS

Wash the buttocks with warm water and soap. Be sure to rinse completely. To prevent diaper rash, it is important to clean the buttocks with soap and water whenever your baby is soiled, not just at bath time. Pay special attention to the creases where matter may collect.

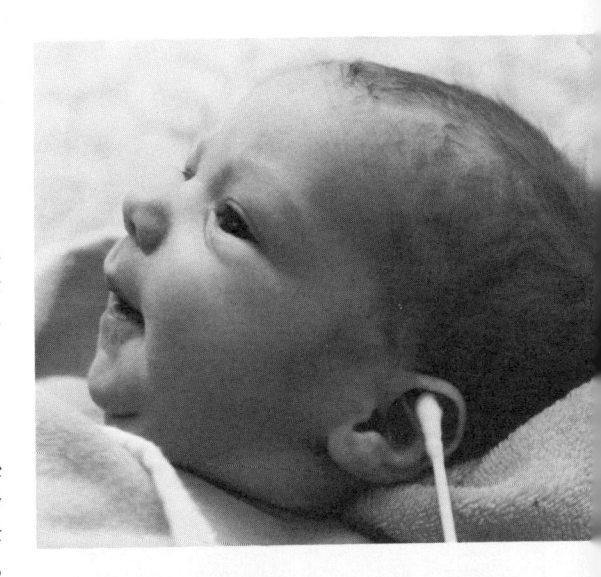

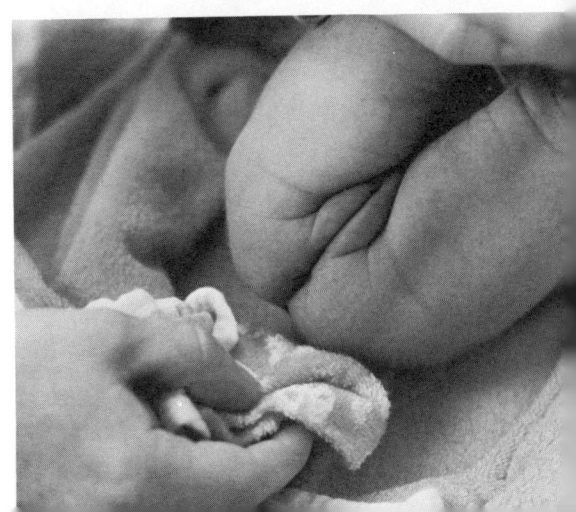

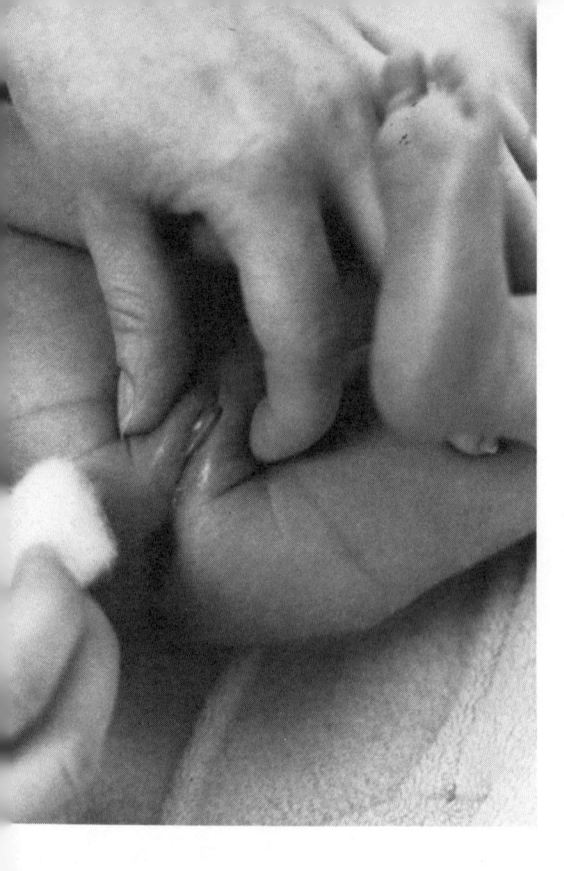

GENITALS

Use a cotton or cloth moistened with water to wash the genitals of a girl. Separate the labia, or lips, and clean down each side from front to back, using a fresh piece of cotton each time.

If your son is circumcised, the foreskin of the penis is removed. The first day, a sterile ointment such as vaseline keeps the area lubricated and helps it to heal. Some doctors suggest that you keep the end of the penis clean with clear water until it is healed. If there is bleeding, call your doctor.

To wash the genital area of a baby boy who is not circumcised, gently push back the foreskin, but only as far as it will go easily. Never force the foreskin. Clean it carefully with cotton moistened in water.

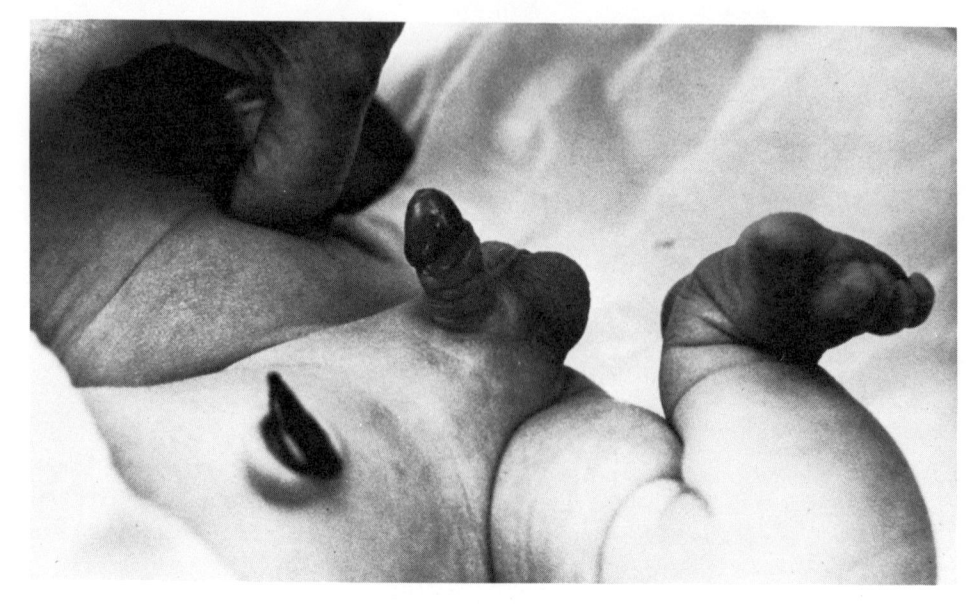

64

UMBILICAL CORD

During pregnancy your baby is attached to the placenta by the umbilical cord. At birth the cord is cut about two inches from your baby's body. It appears as a dry, brownish stump, and causes your baby no pain. The base of the umbilical stump should be cleaned two or three times a day with alcohol until it is completely healed and the stump drops off naturally. A slight amount of bloody drainage may be seen at the time it drops off, about seven to ten days after birth. Using a cotton swab dipped in alcohol, be sure to clean the folds around the cord. There are no nerve endings in the cord so you cannot hurt your baby by handling it. Fold diapers down in front to keep the cord from getting wet, and avoid using rubber pants. Do not immerse your baby in bath water until the cord has fallen off. Call your doctor if you notice bleeding, pus, a bad smell, or a red area in the belly around the base of the stump. The red line where the cord and the future belly button come together is normal, but the belly skin should not be red.

RINSE AND DRY

Because your baby's skin is extremely delicate, it is important that you rinse it well. Dry all the creases carefully, especially where irritation may occur. Use powder sparingly; baby powder has a tendency to cake and irritate and may be inhaled when it is being applied and may interfere with your baby's perspiration system and cause rashes.

OTHER CARE

Diaper Care

Some babies won't tolerate a wet or soiled diaper, while others don't care. As long as your baby does not develop redness or a rash, you are changing his diapers often enough.

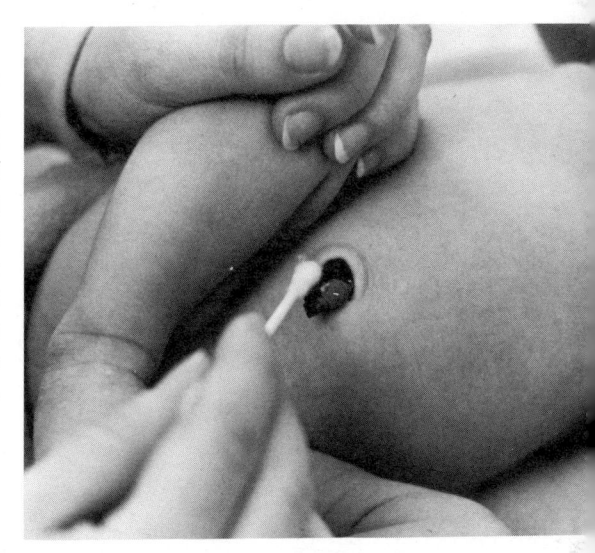

There are a variety of diapers to choose from. You can buy cotton or flannelette diapers, disposable diapers, or disposable liners to use in any diaper. Do not use double diapers, as too much bulk can push your baby's legs and pelvis out of normal alignment. If you are using safety pins, be sure they are always pointed away from your baby.

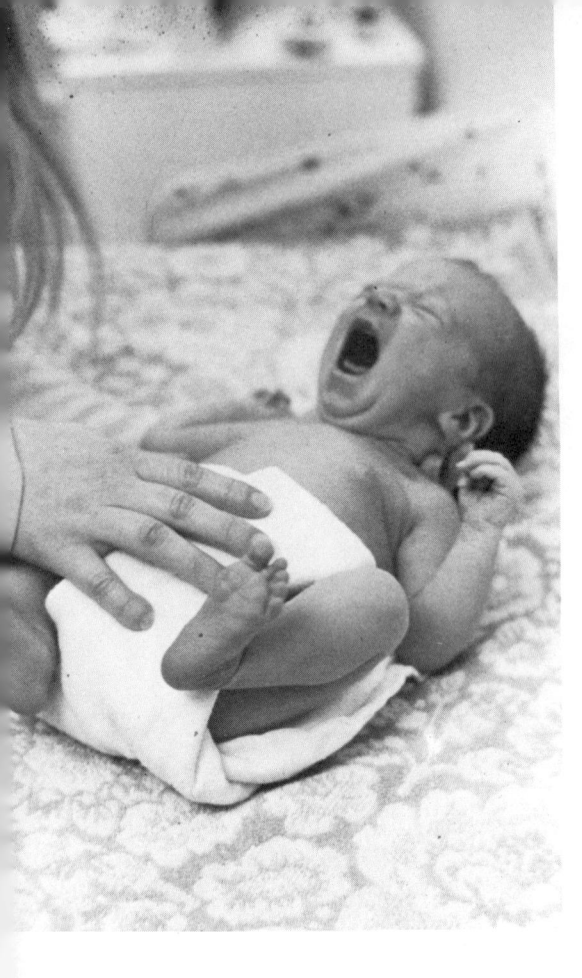

There are a number of ways to fold diapers. For your newborn you may simply want to fold the diaper into a triangle and fasten the three corners in front with a single pin. For extra thickness at the back for a girl and at the front for a boy, you can fold a rectangular diaper into a square, turn the right side in one third, the left side in one third and fold the top over, using a pin to fasten each side.

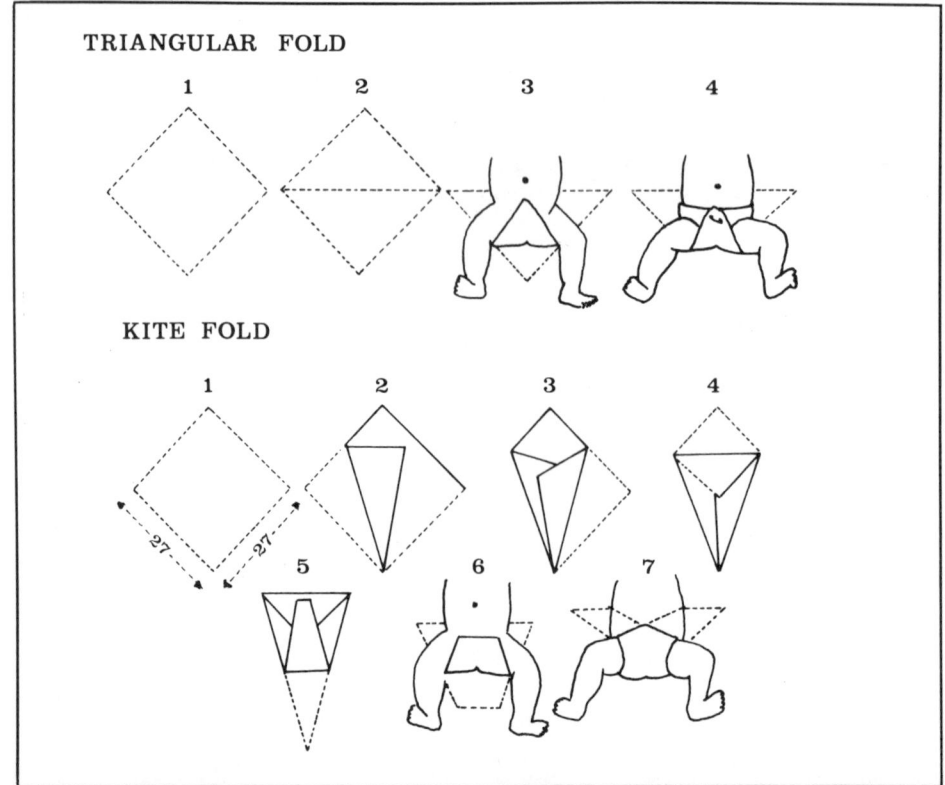

TRIANGULAR FOLD

KITE FOLD

Dressing

Your baby's heat regulating system isn't very efficient at first. When inside, dress him as you dress yourself for warmth. His hands and feet should be cool to the touch, and his body warm. He needs freedom of movement, so don't bundle him too tightly. Protect him from drafts, and keep the room temperature slightly higher than normal.

COLD WEATHER

Babies do not perspire efficiently and can become overheated easily. When you dress your baby in cold weather, dress him as you would yourself. Provide warmth for his legs and feet as well as his head and trunk.

HOT WEATHER

When it is hot, keep your baby in a cool, shady spot with his eyes and head protected. Be careful not to expose your baby to too much sun since he can become seriously sunburned.

SWADDLING

Babies like swaddling—being snuggled warm and secure. Fold down the top of a receiving blanket and place your baby on the upper two-thirds. Fold up the bottom of the triangle. Fold in one side snugly and then the other. Babies like to feel pressure against their tummies.

Exercise

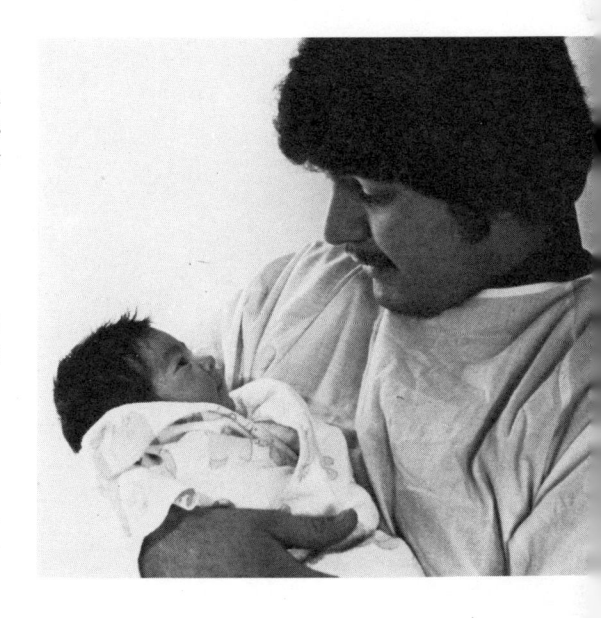

Exercise is important to your new baby. Keep diapers and clothes loose enough so he can move around freely. When your baby is awake, put him on a firm surface and leave him free to move his arms and legs. Beware of overusing infant seats, carriers, Snuglis, or swings. Limited use is fine, but too much will restrict normal arm, leg, and muscle development.

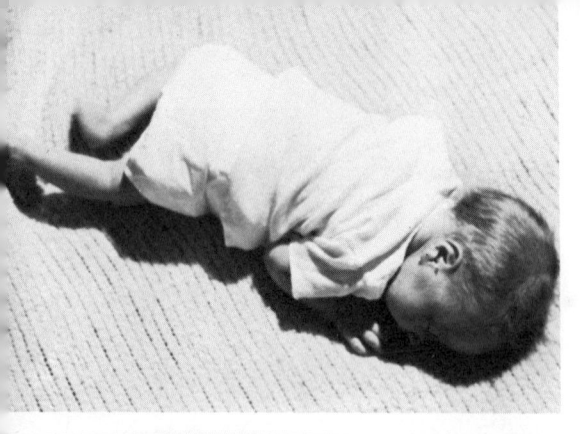

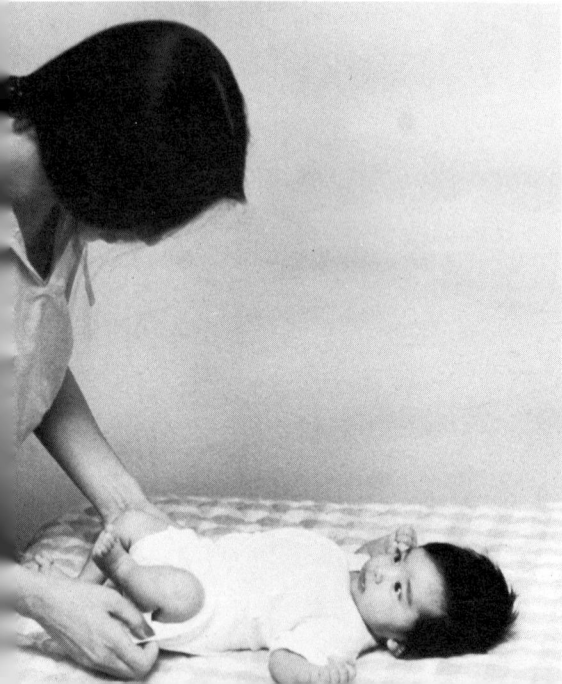

Sunning

Sunshine is healthy for your baby, but be careful of how much. He can be exposed for two to three minutes a day of direct sunlight. Be sure his eyes are shaded.

Sleep

Your baby's sleep is a time for growth and development. Every newborn not only has a unique personality, but also an individual sleeping pattern. After birth it will take him some time to get his system regulated and adjusted to his new existence. He usually spends his first few sleeping times in a restorative sleep. When he comes home it will take him some time to adjust to his new situation there. However, once he gets regulated, the new baby has an average of 7 or 8 sleeping and waking periods each day. Most infants sleep from 12 to 20 hours in a 24-hour day, and are alert only about 30 minutes out of every four hours. During sleep your newborn will stir, twitch, stretch, whimper, grimace, smile, frown, and act startled.

Your baby can sleep in a crib or a bassinet. During the night, many new mothers who are breast-feeding like to have a bassinet close to their beds so that they can just reach over and get their baby for the night feeding. The baby may stay safely in the parents' bed before and after the feeding. (Parents will not roll over and suffocate a baby any more than they would each other.)

CLOTHES AND EQUIPMENT

An important part of preparing for and enjoying your new baby is gathering the clothes and equipment that will make your job more enjoyable. You will be faced with a wide variety of choices. Choose items that are simple, durable, and easy to wash.

Clothes

Essential clothing to get you through the first few months of parenting will include four dozen diapers, six pairs of plastic pants, six undershirts, six kimonos and gowns, three sacque sets, three stretch suits, one sweater and cap, 3 pair socks, booties, and six bibs.

Blankets and Sheets

You will need a minimum of four receiving (lightweight) blankets, a sleeping blanket or sleeper, three crib sheets, three waterproof lap pads, one mattress cover or large pad, two quilted crib pads, and one comforter or quilt.

Bath Equipment

You will need at least two large bath towels, six washclothes, three hand towels, a bathinnet or portable baby bath, a brush and comb, nail scissors, and toiletries, which should include a mild soap, lotion, cornstarch, petroleum jelly, cotton swabs, baby shampoo, rubbing alcohol, safety pins, and cotton balls.

Nursery Equipment

For your baby's comfort you will want a baby crib (a bassinet or basket can be used for a newborn), a mattress, crib bumper, chest of drawers, and laundry hamper. For diapering needs you will want diaper pins, a dressing or changing table, and a diaper pail.

Feeding Equipment

If you are breast-feeding, you will need three bottles for water and juice, and nursing pads. If you are bottle-feeding, you will need eight bottles, nipples, and caps.

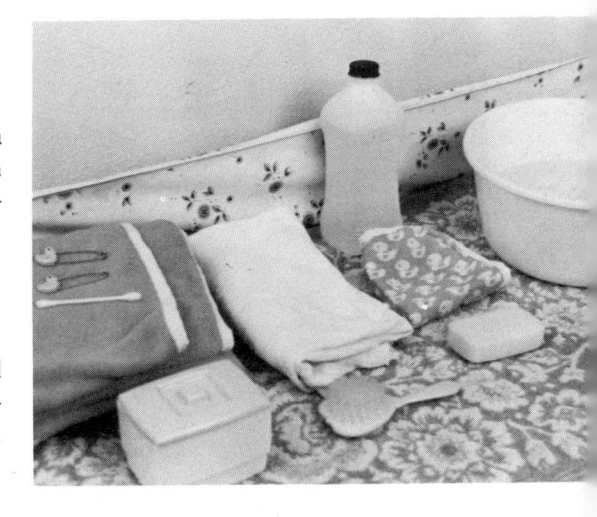

Your Baby's Medicine Cabinet

The following will help you in your baby's care:

- Rectal thermometer
- Hot water bottle
- Mineral oil
- Petroleum jelly
- Baby aspirin (as prescribed by your doctor)
- Sterile cotton
- Antiseptic (for diaper rash, recommended by doctor)
- Soft bulb syringe
- Sterile gauze bandages
- Vaporizer

Optional Equipment

There are many other items that make life more pleasant for baby and mother. Among the most important is a rocking chair. It is wonderful for soothing and relaxing both baby and mother. A front pack or side sling is great for an irritable or crying baby. A backpack is important for baby, mother, and father. Other options include a playpen and an electric bottle warmer.

BABY-SITTERS

Although you will not want to leave your newborn right away, you should be developing baby-sitters you are confident of. Find baby-sitters whose philosophy is consistent with yours, who can care physically for your child, and who are dependable.

1. Try to trade services with your relatives.

2. Ask your neighbors, family, and friends for names of persons who have cared for their babies whom they know and like.
3. Check the want ads and bulletin boards at grocery stores, churches, et cetera. Call the person with a list of questions concerning their experience, philosophy, and dependability. Ask for a personal interview and ask for and follow up on references.
4. Check into baby-sitting cooperatives, usually made up of women who have children about the same age. These may be organized by neighborhood, church, or childbirth groups.
5. Call your local school, university, sorority, fraternity, or other student organization and ask if they have a list of persons interested in baby-sitting. Again, arrange an interview before you hire anyone. Ask for references.
6. There are professional care organizations that advertise in the newspaper or are listed in the yellow pages. Interview persons interested. Ask for references and be sure to follow them up.

TRAVELING WITH YOUR NEWBORN

Although your newborn is a good traveler, during his early days you should not expose him to crowds in small enclosed places, or to people who have any infectious diseases, such as cold or flu. It is good for your baby to get out in the fresh, open air. Your basic problems in traveling with your baby will be feeding and keeping him clean.

Feeding

If you are breast-feeding, you will have no problem meeting his feeding schedule. If you are bottle-feeding, you must plan ahead. If you will be out for only a short time, you can prepare formula ahead of time and take it in an insulated container. If you will be out for a long time, it is better to take prepared canned formula.

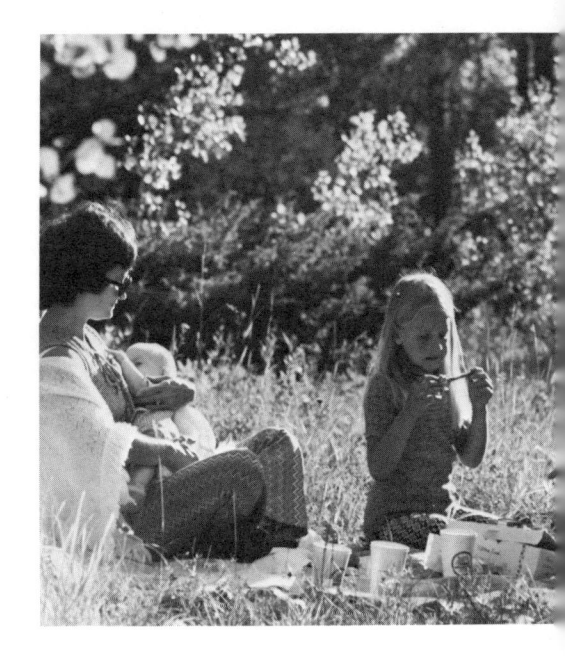

Cleaning

Take along disposable diapers and disposable wipes for changing your baby. Several wet washclothes in a plastic bag will help you clean your baby's face after eating and the soiled diaper area. A plastic bag is good for the soiled diapers.

Carrying

A front pack for your new baby is a comfortable way to take him around. An umbrella stroller is lightweight and easily portable. If your baby will be riding in a car, be sure you invest in an approved car seat for your baby's safety. As your baby grows, a backpack is indispensable for both the mother and the father.

8.

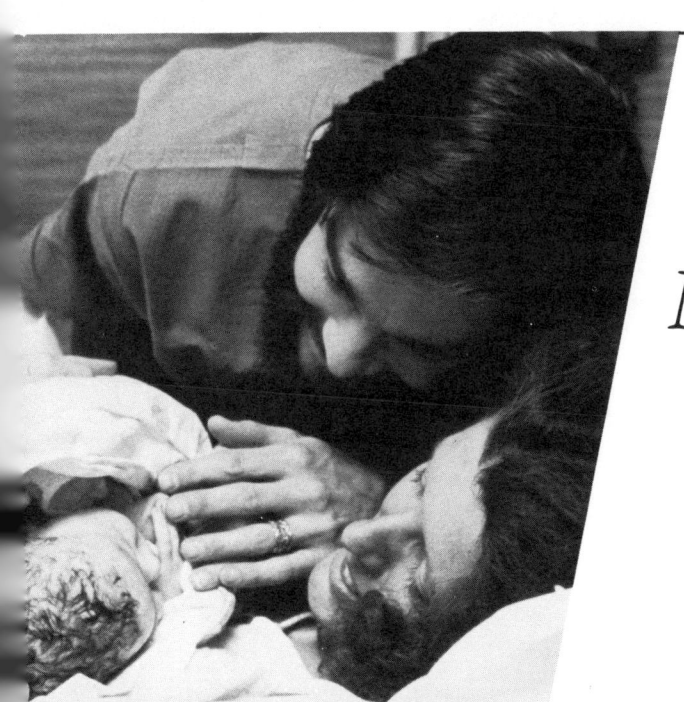

Common Concerns of New Parents

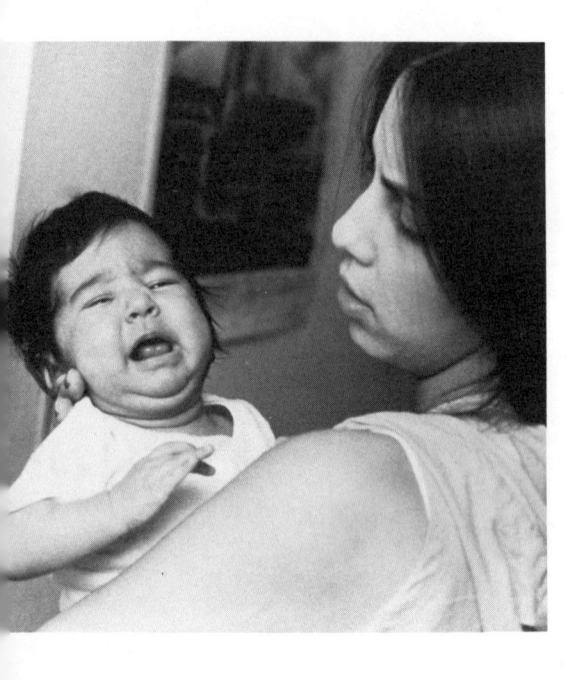

As you hold your new baby in your arms you may become overwhelmed by the size of the task ahead of you. Although feeding, cleaning, soothing, and playing with your baby may seem complex, they will soon become a routine. There will still be unpredictable elements, however, that may give you reason for concern.

CHOOSING YOUR BABY DOCTOR

One of the most important persons to whom you will turn when you are concerned about your baby is your baby's medical caregiver. When selecting a pediatrician, family practitioner, general practitioner, or pediatric nurse practitioner be sure you choose one in whom you have confidence. Be sure to interview and select your caregiver before your baby's birth. Some of the questions you may want answered are:

- Does the doctor make house calls? (Although this is almost never necessary, it is nice to know that you have a doctor you can count on should an emergency arise.)
- What are his/her policies on telephone consultations (will he/she return and answer your calls and is there a charge)?
- What are his/her policies of visiting your baby immediately following birth?
- How does the doctor feel about circumcision and is it compatible with your feelings?
- What are the doctor's feelings about breast-feeding and bottle-feeding and can he or she give you the information and support your need for breast-feeding if you have chosen to nurse your baby?
- Can you call the doctor on the telephone for information and questions when you first bring your baby home?
- What are the doctor's feelings about feeding schedules (fixed routine vs. demand feelings) and are they compatible with yours?
- What are the doctors' policies for prescribing medications (early prescription of medications during illness vs. the natural approach) and are they compatible with yours?

- Who covers for the doctor when he/she is away?
- What hospital will your child be sent to if she is sick? (Be sure the affiliation is with a hospital that you are confident of.)

There are times when your newborn's immature systems cannot send out clear signals whether she is really in trouble or simply enduring a difficult moment. Colic and uncontrolled crying may be your first worry, and there are many other common physical problems that may give you moments of uncertainty.

ELIMINATION

Diarrhea

It is normal for a baby to have loose stools, especially if she is breast-fed or is on a formula whose composition is similar to breast milk. However, if your baby's stools have mucus, are foul smelling, become green, or are expelled with force it may be a sign of diarrhea. Since diarrhea is a symptom of intestinal infection, illness, or irritation, it is important that you call your doctor or clinic for care. Give your baby only boiled water. If you are breast-feeding, continue.

Constipation

It is not uncommon for a baby to go for more than one day without a bowel movement; however, if the stools are hard, dry, and difficult to pass, your baby may be constipated. If your baby is constipated try to increase the fluids in her diet. Although the condition is rare in breast-fed babies, you can increase your own fluid intake to help correct constipation. If it continues for more than a week, or if there is blood in your baby's stools, call your doctor. Never give an enema or laxative unless it is prescribed by your doctor.

EATING PROBLEMS

Spitting Up

It is common for your newborn to spit up surplus milk following a feeding. Spitting up may be caused by swallowing air during a feeding or an immature sphincter muscle at the entrance to the stomach. To minimize the amount of air swallowed in a bottle-fed baby, hold the bottle so that no air is in the nipple. In a breast-fed baby, allow the first stream of milk to spurt into a cup or bottle, and then put your baby to your breast. Burp your baby before, during, and after feedings. Avoid overfeeding and handle your baby gently after her feeding. Not letting your baby cry too long or hard before feedings may also be helpful. As your baby matures, the sphincter muscle becomes stronger and does not allow milk to come up.

It is serious if your baby spits up in a forceful or projectile type of vomiting. Contact your doctor.

Hiccups

Your baby probably had hiccups in the uterus and may have frequent attacks after eating. Although they can be quite disconcerting to you, they don't seem to bother your baby. Try giving her a little sip of water or changing her position.

RASHES

Cradle Cap

Your baby may have what look like flakes, scales, or crusty material on her head. If you find after daily washing and brushing that it persists, call your doctor for suggestions.

Facial Rashes

Various facial rashes—small red spots, rough spots, and small pimples—are common for all infants during the first few months. Small white spots on your baby's nose, cheeks, and chin are obstructed sweat and oil glands. Red streaks on her neck, eyelids, nose, or forehead are superficial blood vessels. All these facial markings eventually fade and disappear.

Prickly Heat

If your baby is overdressed during warm weather, she may develop a rash on her shoulder and neck regions. A light application of cornstarch may help. Prickly heat can be prevented by keeping your baby cool and dry.

Diaper Rash

If your baby develops diaper rash, don't be alarmed. Diaper rash is a red rash in your baby's genital area that varies in severity. It is caused by the ammonia and bacteria in the baby's urine or the burning effect of the bowel movement on your baby's skin. Be sure to change diapers frequently, and clean your baby with soap and water each time she is soiled. Rince completely and dry well. Apply A & D or Desitin ointment to promote healing and prevent further burn from urine. Expose your baby's bottom to air two or three times a day. Wash the diapers away from other laundry. Soak them in a solution of one tablespoon vinegar to three quarts water, use a mild soap to wash, and rinse three times to get all of the soap out. Hang the diapers in bright sunlight if possible.

Thrush

Thrush, caused by a fungus, looks like patches of milk curds on the roof of your baby's mouth, tongue, and the insides of her cheeks. It causes your baby's mouth to be sore and makes it difficult for her to nurse. Call your doctor or clinic immediately for care. Giving your baby sterile water to drink after each feeding may give her some relief.

Eczema

Eczema is a rough, scaly, red, itchy rash in a distinct small area. It is a common allergic reaction in babies and can be caused by food, clothing, or anything that comes in contact with your baby's skin. Contact your doctor or clinic for ointments and treatment.

WHEN TO CALL YOUR DOCTOR

Every mother experiences moments when her baby is not feeling well. You know your baby better than anyone, and when she is not herself you know it right away. However, sometimes it is difficult to decide when your baby's symptoms are severe enough to call your doctor. Below are some guidelines to follow, but whenever you are extremely worried, it's best to call your doctor right away simply to relieve your mind.

Have faith in your instinct and common sense. A slight temperature or a mild cold usually do not need medical help. But if you see the following behavioral or physical changes in your baby, let your doctor or clinic help guide you in your baby's care. When you call, be sure to tell them what you have done in the way of food, medications, or any other treatment and how your baby responded.

Behavior Changes

- Excessive crying: You know when your baby's crying means she is irritable or has colic. When her crying is excessive and her appearance and color seem different, she may be sick.
- Unusual irritability: crying combined with a high degree of irritability that is not your baby's usual state, along with restlessness.
- Changed sleeping patterns: excessive drowsiness or unusually poor sleep patterns with waking and crying periods.
- Appetite: loss of appetite and continuous refusal to take food.
- Movement: listlessness, restlessness, and thrashing about.

WHAT TO TELL YOUR DOCTOR

PHYSICAL CHANGES (*How Your Baby Looks*)	BEHAVIOR CHANGES (*How Your Baby Acts*)
My baby's temperature is _____ .	My baby is crying: (excessively, high-pitched).
My baby's skin is: (flushed, hot, dry, pale).	My baby's behavior is: (irritable, restless, miserable).
My baby has vomited: (between feedings, a large part of her feeding, with unusual force).	My baby's sleeping is: (prolonged, intermittent).
	My baby's appetite is: (poor, nonexistent).
My baby's bowel movements are: (color, consistency, odor and frequency).	My baby's movement is: (listless, restless, thrashing).
My baby is: (coughing, sneezing, hoarse).	
My baby's breathing is: (noisy, difficult, rapid, slow).	
My baby's eyes are: (irritated, inflamed, discharging).	
My baby's movements are: (abnormal, twitching, stiff, convulsed).	

Physical Changes

- Elevated temperature: When your baby has a temperature of 101°F. or more (98.6°F. is considered normal), she may have a fever (although babies often run a high temperature simply as a result of lots of activity).
- Skin changes: When your baby has a flushed face, hot or dry skin, or is perspiring, or if she is pale and listless, she may be sick even though her temperature is normal.
- Repeated vomiting, in which your baby throws up most of her feedings.
- Diarrhea: Stools that are watery or contain pus or blood, with loose, frequent bowel movements.
- Inflammation or discharge from the eyes (although some babies develop a mild inflammation of the eye because of a blocked tear duct that is not serious).

- Coughing, severe hoarseness, or a stuffy nose that causes difficulty in breathing.
- Convulsions: If your baby has a relatively high fever, she may experience convulsions. Although frightening, they are seldom dangerous and are usually over in a few minuttes. Call your doctor immediately.
- Pain: When your baby cries in a high-pitched tone and is inconsolable, call your doctor.

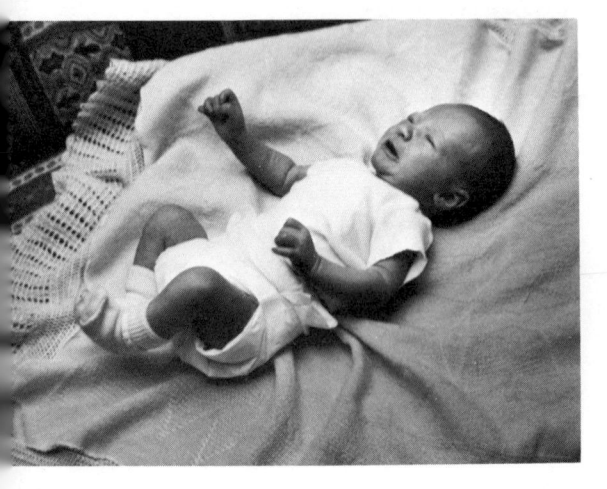

WHEN YOUR BABY IS SICK

Sleep and rest are important when your baby is ill. Keep the room quiet and dark and keep her away from people. Forget feeding and sleeping schedules and let her rest as much as possible. If your baby has a cough or stuffy nose, keep the room humid and warm, but not overheated.

If your baby has a fever, don't urge her to eat. When she is awake, offer her liquids or milk every half hour. If your baby vomits, let her stomach rest. Don't try to feed her, but give her some sterile water. If the water stays down and she wants more, give her a little at a time.

Use medication only when and in the amount your doctor prescribes. Give an enema only when it is prescribed. Do not use leftover prescriptions; throw any leftovers away.

If your baby has a fever, sponging or a wet rub may help to lower your baby's temperature. With a cool wet sponge rub each of your baby's arms, then each leg and finally her back. Take a few minutes to stroke each part.

Remember that when your baby is sick, she needs not only your physical help, but your sympathy, tenderness, and love.

9.

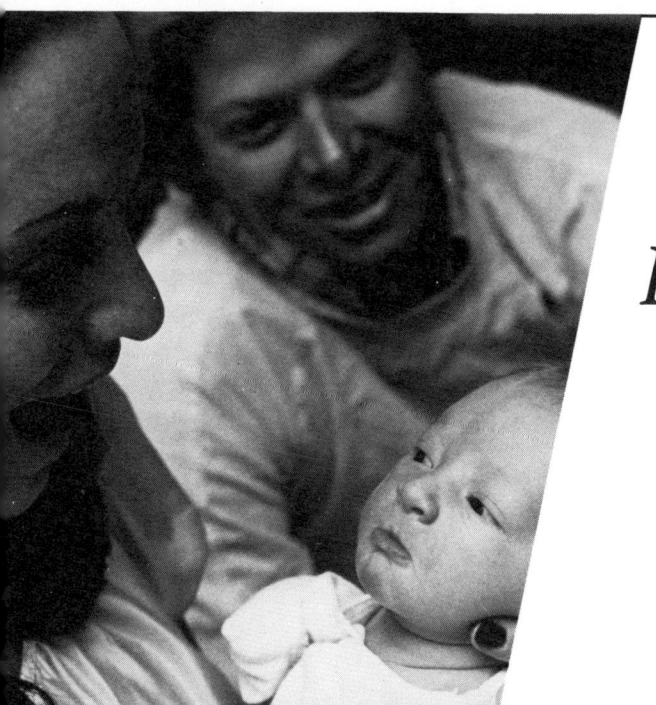

Mother's Recovery After Delivery

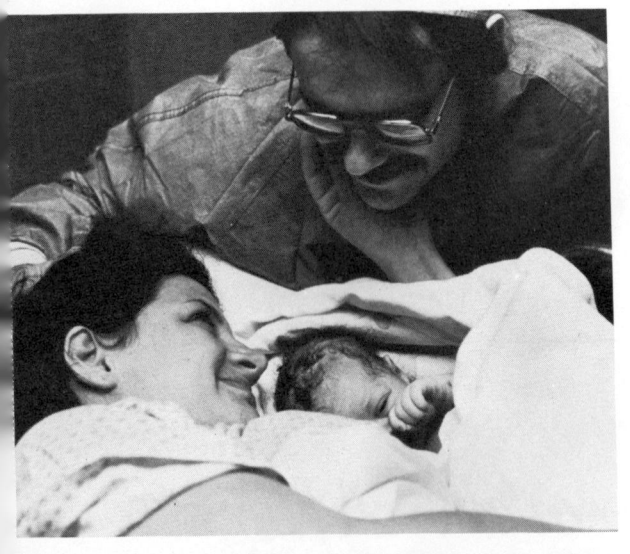

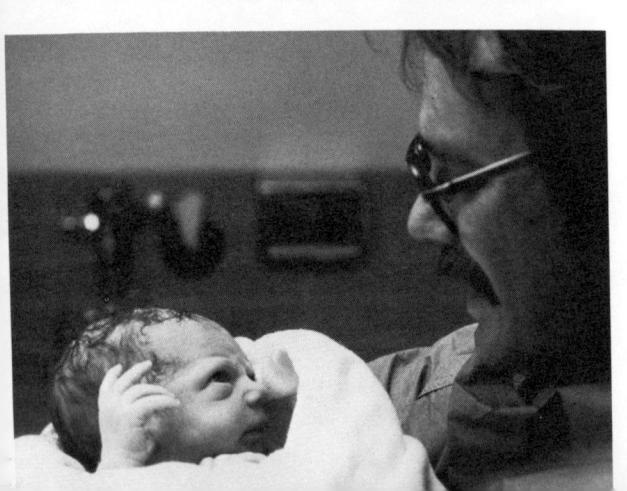

The postpartum period starts with the end of labor and lasts for six to eight weeks. It marks the end of pregnancy and the beginning of parenthood. The postpartum period is an integral part of childbirth and is almost as miraculous as pregnancy itself. The mother's body needs special care as it returns to its nonpregnant condition. There is no other time when your body's organs and systems undergo such rapid and traumatic change.

DELIVERY

At the birth of your baby, it is normal to experience feelings of great joy, satisfaction, and pride. You both may wish to relive the birth over and over and to touch and watch your baby.

The father may experience great feelings of responsibility and protectiveness toward mother and baby. You, the mother, may feel vulnerable and uncertain about your mothering skills, and you may begin to experience a wide range of feelings, from elation to deep depression.

Placenta

Following delivery, shrinking of your empty uterus causes the placenta to detach from the wall of the uterus. Within a few minutes, your uterus expels the placenta—now no longer needed as your baby's lifeline of nourishment and oxygen.

Your doctor checks your cervix and vagina to make sure no injury occurred during delivery. If you had an episiotomy, the incision is closed with stitches. Although a local anesthetic is usually given for this, you may feel a pricking sensation.

Your uterus continues to contract and relax to control bleeding where the placenta was attached. Since bleeding is always a concern after birth, sustained contraction of your uterus is important in preventing hemorrhaging. Massage and pressure on your uterus is important, even though it may be uncomfortable. Medication may be given immediately after the placenta is delivered, or your baby may be put to your breast on the delivery table to stimulate uterine contractions.

THE CRITICAL FIRST HOUR

You are carefully observed for an hour after the birth. During this time, your attendant is especially concerned with the condition of your uterus, vagina, and perineum, and with your body's reaction to the trauma of labor and delivery. You are checked every 15 minutes during this hour for any complications.

Uterus

The attendant examines your uterus by placing the side of her hand on top of and slightly cupped under the uterus, while her other hand is placed over your pubic bone with light pressure. If she finds that it is not firm, she massages your uterus until it contracts.

She also examines the area just above your pubic arch for any stretching of your bladder. If it is full, or filling, a bulge will be evident. Since a full bladder could inhibit uterine contractions, she may consider using a catheter to draw off the urine. At the same time, she presses blood and clots from the uterus every 15 minutes for the first hour and every 30 minutes for the second hour to ensure that your uterus stays firm. The first hour after childbirth you bleed about as much as you would for a heavy menstrual period. The blood is bright red and fresh.

Blood Pressure and Pulse Rate

Your blood pressure and pulse rate are checked as an indication of how well your body is recovering. If a large amount of blood has been lost, your circulatory system will probably not be able to compensate and a rapid increase in your pulse rate and abrupt drop in your blood pressure may occur.

Shaking and Chattering

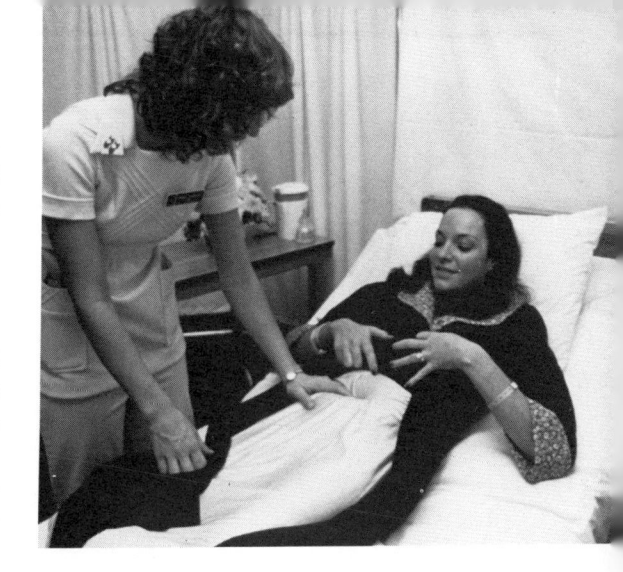

You may experience shaking, chattering teeth, and trembling limbs while still in the recovery room. Use your slow chest breathing and try to relax. A warm blanket feels especially good. This will last only a short time.

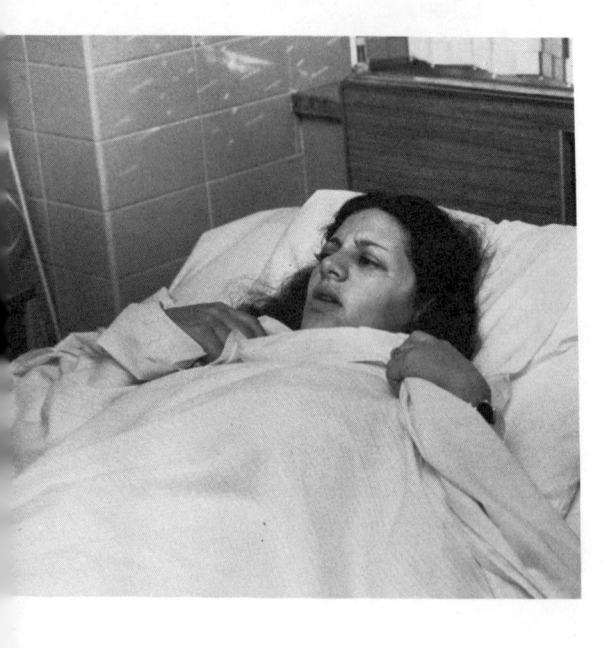

FIRST DAYS

Uterus

The first day after childbirth, your uterus should feel like a firm mass about the size of a grapefruit in the middle of your abdomen. It is probably about three finger widths, or 1½ inches, below your navel. Feel it periodically and massage it gently if it is not firm and low in your abdomen. If it will not stay firm, contact your doctor. In the next few weeks the size of your uterus diminishes until, in about a week, it is difficult to find. As you nurse your baby, you feel mild cramps. These keep your uterus well contracted.

Bleeding

Be sure someone is with you when you get out of bed for the first time; you may feel faint. Blood can pool in your vagina during your rest period, and you may experience a gush of blood when you stand up.

By the third day, your bleeding has decreased and become lighter in color. By the tenth day the discharge, called lochia, is often pale yellow, sticky, and watery. If, at any time, you thoroughly wet two pads in one hour, or the discharge smells foul or continues to be bright red after the first day, be sure to contact your doctor.

Stitches

The stitches of an episiotomy usually are absorbed or drop out as your incision heals. There may be pain or itching during the healing process. Using a heat lamp or taking sitz baths may reduce the pain. Apply an ice pack to reduce swelling. If pain is severe and persistent, tell your caregiver. Complete, firm healing of the episiotomy may take several weeks.

Cleanliness

It is important to keep the area between the vagina and the anus clean. Anything that enters your vagina can infect the wall of your uterus where the placenta was attached. Your stitches and episiotomy are also open to infection. Clean your perineum after going to the bathroom and when changing your sanitary pads. You may want to pour warm water over the area. Be sure to wipe from front to back to prevent spreading bacteria from your rectum to your vagina. Use sterile sanitary pads, touching only the ends, and change them frequently.

Elimination/Urination

Pressure on your bladder during pregnancy and delivery coupled with the effects of local anesthetics lessen your awareness of a full bladder and your ability to start the flow of urine. Although you may have difficulty in the first few hours after delivery, it is important to void as soon as possible and as often as necessary to keep your bladder empty. A full bladder makes it difficult for the uterus to stay contracted. It's normal to pass large amounts of urine after delivery.

Bowel Movement

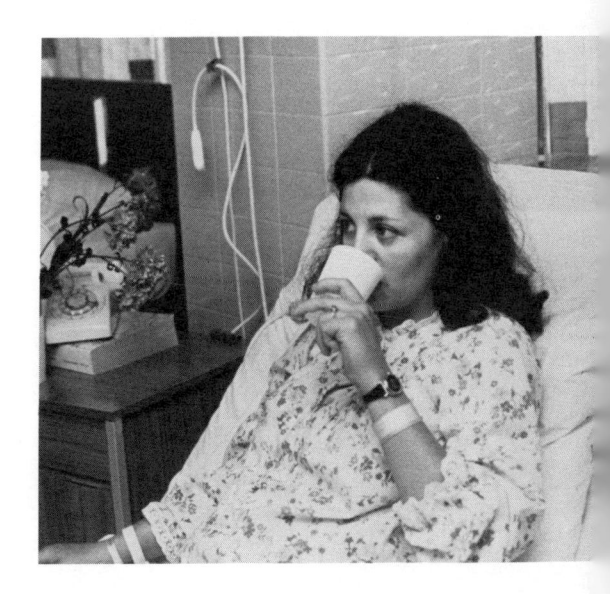

Be sure to drink plenty of fluids and eat a well-balanced diet that includes lots of roughage. You should have a bowel movement within two to three days after delivery. Constipation can sometimes be a problem in the early days of postpartum. Often the problem is fear of harm to your stitches. But your first bowel movement usually causes you far less discomfort than you anticipate. It is important for you to reestablish normal bowel patterns as soon as possible. Your nurses will be asking daily whether you have had a bowel movement, because this is such an important aspect of your recovery.

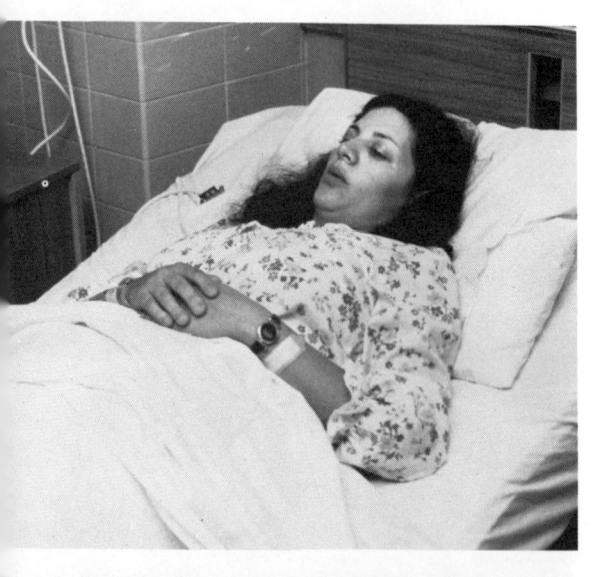

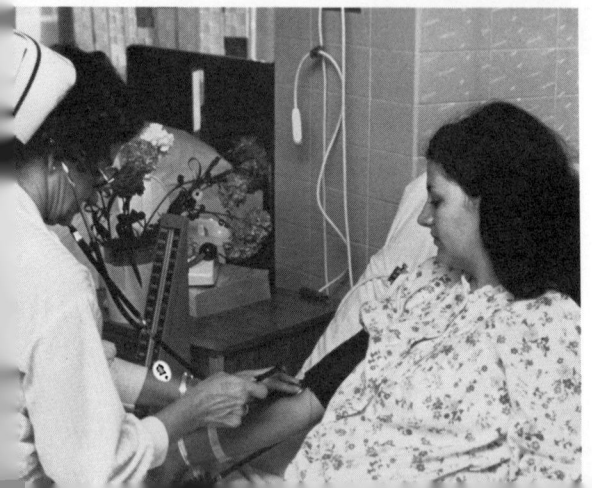

Hemorrhoids

Hemorrhoids may start to bother you at this time, particularly if you have had problems before, or if they are aggravated by the pressure of pushing during delivery. Be sure to tell your attendant if you start to develop hemorrhoids. Sitz baths, suppositories, and cold compresses can all be helpful.

Afterpains

Afterpains are caused by the contractions that return your uterus to its normal condition. They tend to be more pronounced when your baby is being breast-fed. Afterpains occur less frequently with your first baby, and are more intense with subsequent births. In some instances afterpains may continue for several days and occasionally are severe enough to require medication. Concentration on deep breathing and relaxation may help you handle the discomforts of afterpains.

Monitoring

Because the uterus is raw at the point where your placenta was attached, it is important to guard against infection until the healing is well underway. Your blood pressure, pulse, and temperature are all indications of how well the healing is progressing, so they are checked daily.

Weight Gain and Loss

The weight you have gained results from both the growth of your baby and changes in your own body. Your baby adds approximately eight pounds to your total weight. The placenta adds another pound, and the amniotic fluid, two more. Your breasts each enlarge by about 1 pound and your uterus by 2 pounds. The increase in your blood volume adds about 3 more pounds. The buildup of fat and fluids adds another 6 or more pounds, giving a minimum weight gain of 24 pounds. At your baby's birth, you lose the weight of your baby, the placenta, and the amniotic fluid. The average new mother still weighs about 13 to 19 pounds extra one hour after delivery. In the following six to eight weeks you gradually lose the fat and fluids that were stored to provide energy for the growth of your baby.

Weight Gain

	pounds
blood volume	3
breasts	2
placenta	1
amniotic fluid	2
uterus	2
baby	8
fats & fluids	6
total	24-30

Skeletal/Muscular

During pregnancy your center of balance shifted, your muscles stretched, your ligaments softened, and your joints loosened. The rate of postpartum recovery depends a great deal on the care you gave your body during pregnancy.

Digestive

Your digestive system is displaced by your growing baby during pregnancy. In your postpartum period the digestive system makes a rapid return to its normal state.

Cardiovascular

Great demands were made on your cardiovascular system during pregnancy. The amount of blood in your body increased from about 5 quarts to approximately 7. In response to this greater load, your heart enlarged and its rate increased during the last months of pregnancy. Most of these changes will be reversed within the first two weeks of postpartum.

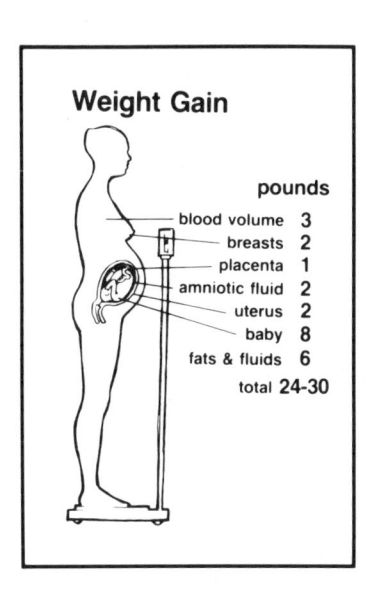

Hormonal

The hormones estrogen and progesterone played a vital role in your pregnancy. They affected your skeletal, muscular, and metabolic functions as well as your emotional base. During postpartum, marked and rapid hormonal changes may have an effect on your emotional balance.

Nervous System

During early postpartum your nervous system may be unstable. Small annoyances may produce anger and emotional upheaval. You need emotional as well as physical rest during the postpartum period.

Elimination

Between the second and fifth days postpartum, your body eliminates more than 2 quarts of extra fluid. Together with the perspiring that may occur, this results in a weight loss of about 5 pounds.

Abdominal Muscles

Delivery will leave your abdomen soft and flabby. As a result of the prolonged extension of the abdominal walls, these muscles remain flabby for some time. Returning them to normal requires at least six weeks. Postnatal exercises may be started during the first week, then gradually increased.

Skin

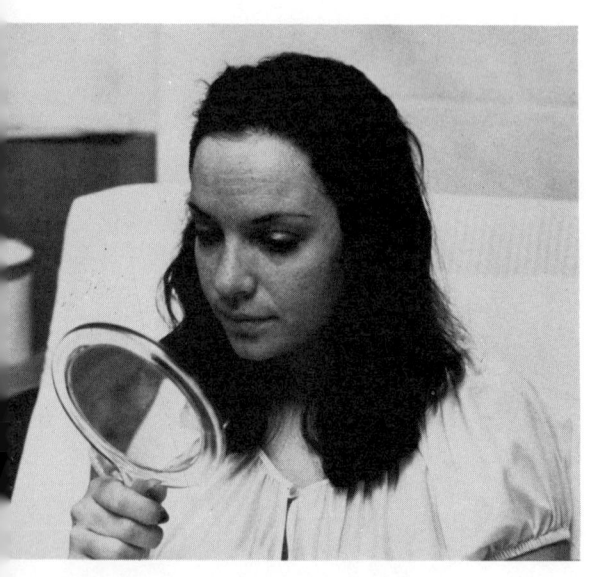

As your pregnancy progressed, the skin of your abdomen stretched and you may have developed slightly purplish stretch marks and lines. These marks eventually fade, although they never completely disappear. Irregular brown spots or blotches, called the "mask of pregnancy," may have appeared on your face. You may have increased pigmentation on your breasts and abdomen. These changes in your skin are due to the stresses caused by the growth of your baby and to deposits of pigments caused by hormones. Except for stretch marks, most of these skin changes disappear soon after your baby's birth.

Breasts

Dramatic changes occur in your breasts almost immediately after your baby is born. The earliest milk, colostrum, produced during the latter part of your pregnancy, increases in the first three or four days after delivery. Colostrum is easy for babies to digest. It is rich in minerals and proteins and carries some of your immunities to disease as well as a laxative substance helpful to your newborn. From the second to the fourth day, your breasts become fuller, firmer, and heavier. If you are not nursing, this may cause some discomfort, since it signals the onset of lactation, or the production of milk.

Uterus

Your uterus changed in weight and size during pregnancy: from 2½ ounces to 2½ pounds and from 2 to 12 inches long. It also increased in volume more than 500 times. This amazing growth is the result of new muscle cells and the thickening and lengthening of the muscles of the uterus. After your baby is born, your uterus is about 20 times its normal size. By the end of the first week, your uterus shrinks in size and weighs about one pound. It returns to its original size and weight by the end of the postpartum period.

Cervix

The cervix is the lower part of your uterus that opens into the vagina. During the last weeks of pregnancy, hormones soften its tissues. In labor, the contractions of the uterine muscles draw up the cervix into the body of the uterus and then open it to the size of the baby's head. Immediately after birth the cervix and lower uterus are soft, flabby, collapsed tissues. The opening contracts slowly and closes by the end of the first week.

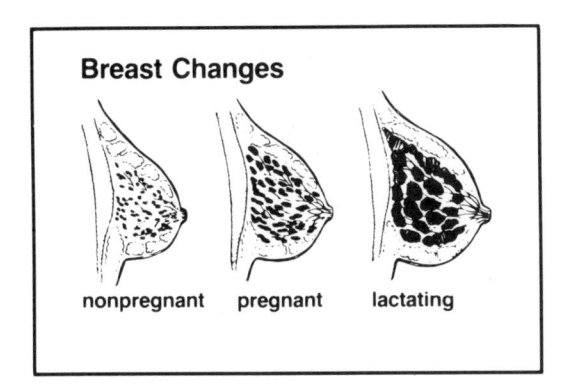

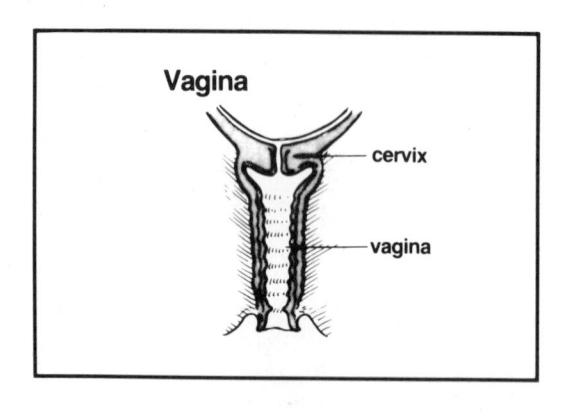

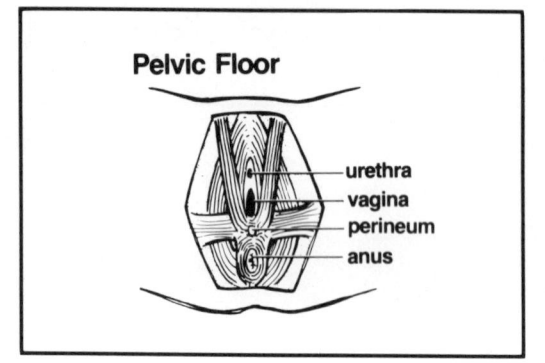

Vagina

Your vagina expanded to allow passage of your baby's head, and then of his body. This passageway is normally 3-5 inches long with walls arranged in thick, expandable folds. Thus your vagina can enlarge to many times its original size for the delivery of your baby. It requires time to recover from this stretching. During postpartum, your vagina gradually diminishes in size.

Pelvic Floor

At birth, your baby passed through the band of muscles, known as the pelvic floor, that forms a sling across the bottom of your pelvis. As your baby's head pushed on your pelvic floor, the muscles were displaced. Other muscles and ligaments in the pelvic regions were also stretched and weakened by your baby's passage through the birth canal. There are special pelvic floor exercises to help firm up these muscles (see Chapter 11, Postnatal Exercises).

ROOMING IN

If you have delivered in a birthing center, your baby will remain with you from birth. However, if your baby is born in a traditional hosptial, with a labor and delivery room, you may have the option of "rooming in" after the birth of your baby.

With rooming in, you have complete care of your baby when he is with you, with a nursing staff available to answer your questions and help you with your baby's care. Rooming in allows you and your baby special time to learn to know one another during the important first days. Your baby spends most of his waking and sleeping time in your room. This time allows you to get to know your baby, his individual rhythms and his unique needs. When you go home you are taking a familiar friend, not a stranger who has been expertly cared for by nurses.

Although with rooming-in service some hospitals leave you and your baby together 24 hours, and only take your baby when you request it, other hospitals will return your

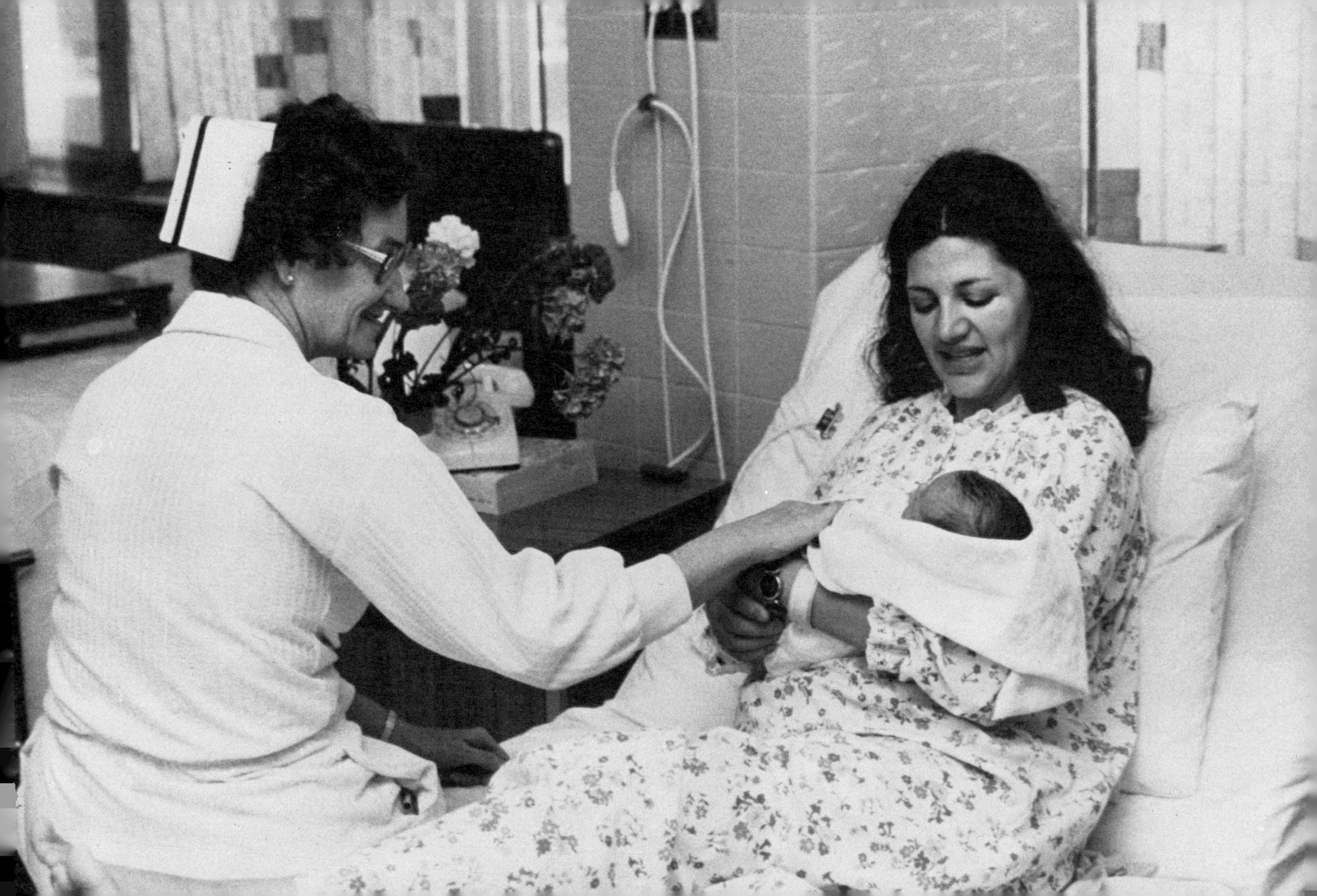

baby to the nursery for the night (from 10:00 P.M. to 8:00 A.M.) and bring him to you for his night feeding. If you have had a long and arduous labor, you may appreciate the nursery taking your baby at night, leaving you to sleep.

With rooming in, you, the father, are considered a part of the family and may visit, hold, and feed your baby. You may be asked to put on a "sterile" gown when you come in. Some hospitals will allow no other visitors in the room with the baby, not even grandparents. If they wish to see the mother, the baby is sent to the nursery or the mother is allowed to visit them in another room.

Rooming in has both advantages and disadvantages. It is important to check with your hospital to see what their policies are. Some of the advantages are:

- The emotional benefits to you and your baby.
- The information and familiarity that rooming in allows you with your newborn.
- A smoother transition from hospital to home for you and your baby.
- You, the father, are allowed to care for and get to know your newborn.
- It helps the breast-feeding mother and newborn develop the breast-feeding process.
- If you have other children at home, this may be the only time you will have alone with this baby.
- In some hospitals, rooming in is less expensive because you do not have to pay for nursery care and personnel.

Some of the disadvantages of rooming in are:

- If you have had a long, hard labor you may need time to recuperate physically.
- If you have other children at home, you may wish to use this time for rest and relaxation.
- In some hospitals, and with some insurance plans, rooming in may be more expensive.
- In some hospitals you are not allowed visitors with rooming in.

10.

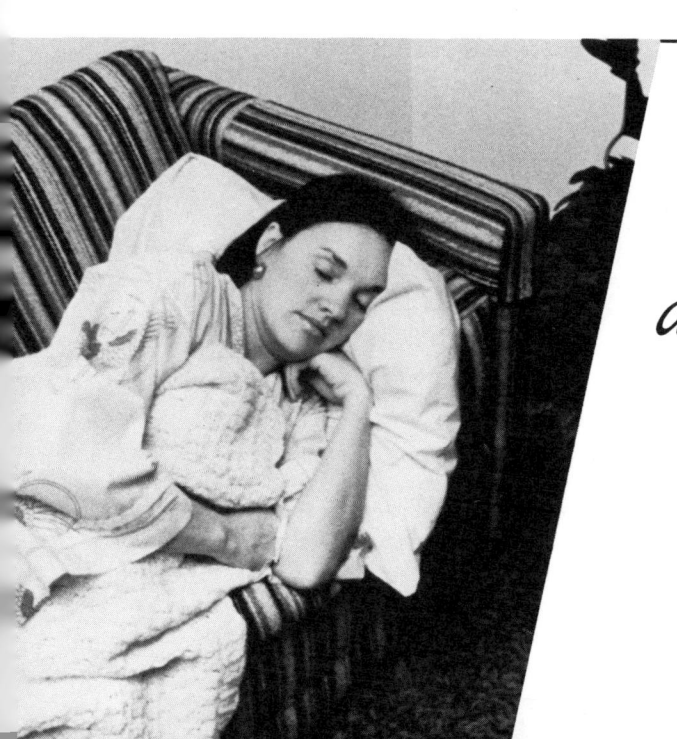

At Home—Daily Care and Nutrition

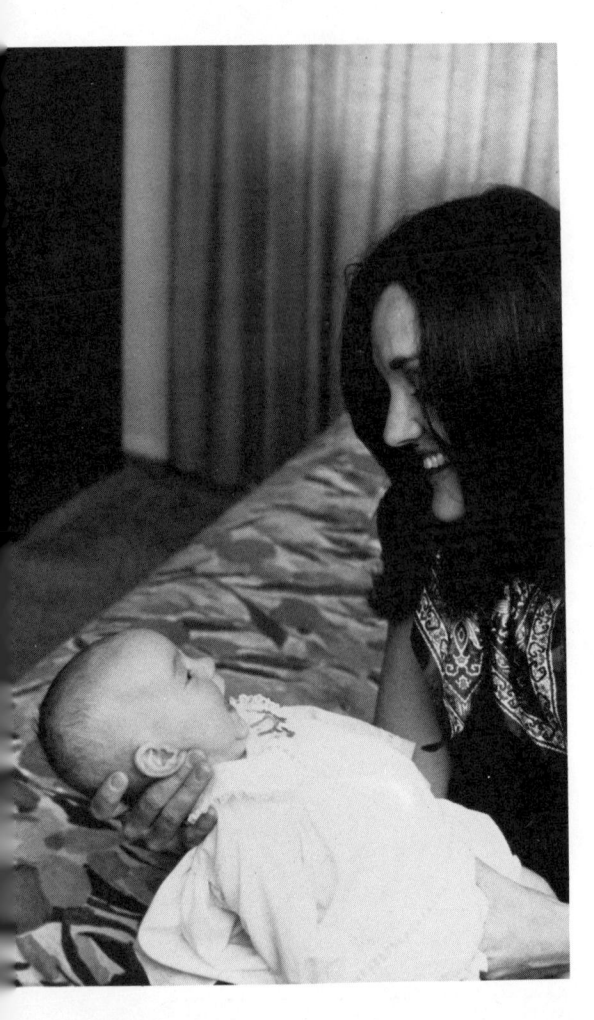

DAILY CARE

Your most difficult time may be the first week at home. You are likely to keep a constant vigil over your newborn baby, and at the same time, in addition to having a house to run, you are concerned with your own physical recovery. Your uterus will shrink to its normal size during the next six weeks, but overactivity can slow this crucial process.

Don't force yourself to do too much too early. Think of the first weeks of postpartum as a birthday present for you and your baby. Take time each day to care for your baby. It will make you feel and look better.

Bathing

Be sure to ask advice about bathing from your own doctor or attendant before you go home. They may suggest a shower for the first few days, waiting until you are fully recovered for a full tub bath. If you have discomfort from your stitches or hemorrhoids, you may find it helpful to take a sitz bath in four inches of warm water three times a day.

Shampooing

Shampoo and set your hair as often as you need. This will keep you looking well and will keep up your spirits.

Perineal Care

To prevent infection and promote healing in the area between your anus and vagina if you have had an episiotomy, sponge the area after each elimination with a mild antiseptic solution. Stitches from your episiotomy will dissolve and your incision is usually healed in less than four weeks. Try whatever comfort measures you used in the hospital to give you relief (sitz baths, cold compresses, heat lamps).

Breast Care

If you are breast-feeding, it is important that you wear a well-fitted bra for comfort and support. Wash your hands before feeding your baby. You can clean the nipple with water (never alcohol) after the feeding. Although your milk will not come in for two or three days after your baby's birth, when it does you will notice your breasts becoming firmer and more engorged as the milk ducts are used for the first time. Engorgement can be relieved by cold packs between feedings and hot packs to enhance the let down right before you feed your baby. Frequent extensive nursing can help relieve the pain and swelling. Pain or streaks of red on your breast signals infection and you must report it immediately to your nurse or attendant.

If you are not breast-feeding you will be given medication to suppress lactation. However, your breasts may become swollen and uncomfortable anyway. Drink less fluid and put cold packs on the breasts.

Vaginal Discharge

You will experience vaginal discharge for as long as four weeks. Because the placental site and the perineal areas are open to infection it is important that you do not douche or use tampons before consulting your doctor or attendant. If the bleeding becomes darker or more profuse, it is a sign that you are doing too much and must rest more.

Menstruation

If you are not breast-feeding, menstruation may return any time after the first month and most probably will come within eight weeks. The first period is likely to seem abnormal. The flow may be heavy and prolonged or scanty and intermittent. Your second period should be more normal. If you are breast-feeding, your first period may occur as early as the second month or as late as eighteen months after delivery. It is likely to be delayed relatively longer if you are feeding your baby only breast milk, with no supplemental fluids or formula, and if you do not give your baby a pacifier.

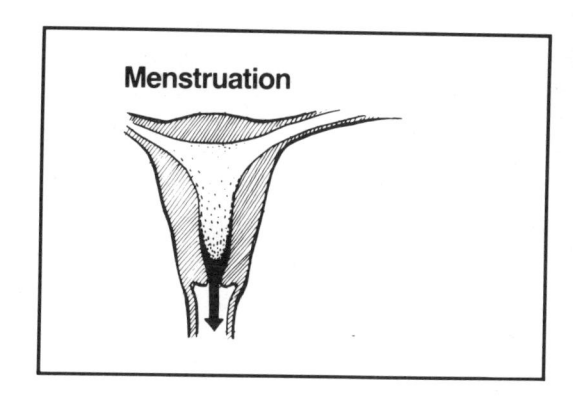

You can nurse during your period. Whether bottle- or breast-feeding, remember that even before your period begins you can ovulate and conceive another baby. So you will want to discuss contraceptives and make your choice before you resume intercourse. If you are breast-feeding, you cannot use birth control pills.

Uterine Cramps

During your postpartum period, contractions will continue to help your uterus return to its normal size within six weeks. If this is your first birth you may not feel them; if it is a subsequent birth, they may become quite uncomfortable. If you are breast-feeding you will probably feel them as your baby sucks at the breast. Try to relax as much as possible and use deep breathing techniques. If they become extremely uncomfortable, ask your doctor, nurse, or attendant for advice.

Constipation

Because of the relaxed state of your abdominal muscles and the soreness of your pelvic floor, you may continue to experience some degree of constipation during the first weeks of postpartum. Be sure you eat lots of fruit, vegetables, whole-grain bread, and cereal. Drink at least eight glasses of water or juice daily. Make a habit of going to the toilet the same time every day. Don't put off having a bowel movement when you feel the urge to do so, but try to establish a regular pattern and time for it. Be sure to get plenty of fresh air and exercise. Should the problem persist, do not self-medicate; consult your doctor.

Hemorrhoids

If you suffered from hemorrhoids during pregnancy you will want to take special care during this postpartum period. Try to avoid constipation by drinking plenty of liquids and eating a balanced diet. Your doctor or caretaker may prescribe medication.

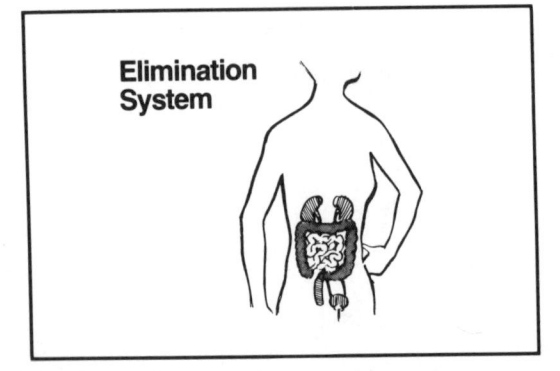

Skin

If you had an increase in skin pigmentation or hair growth during pregnancy you will see it gradually diminishing or fading away. Because you may experience more perspiration it is important that you cleanse your skin daily, using light moisturizers and makeup so you do not clog the pores. Although you may find that baby care and housework leave you little time, the extra effort it takes to keep yourself well groomed will help you feel and look better.

Teeth

Whether you are breast-feeding or not, it is important that you always take special care of your teeth and gums. Brush and floss your teeth every day. If you have put off seeing your dentist during pregnancy, be sure to call and make an appointment for the next month.

Clothing

You will probably be disappointed that you do not fit directly into your prepregnancy wardrobe. Do not become discouraged. Remember, it will take your body at least four to six weeks to lose the extra fluids it stored for your pregnancy. If you can, splurge and buy one outfit that you look and feel good in. You may want to alter your maternity clothes (if you can stand them). Wear your husband's shirts over your maternity pants. And above all, remember that it just takes time.

Smoking

When you were pregnant, if you smoked a cigarette, your baby smoked too. Recent research shows that the lungs of people who live with a heavy smoker look as if they smoked lightly themselves. So, if you must smoke, do it away from your baby and never smoke while feeding her.

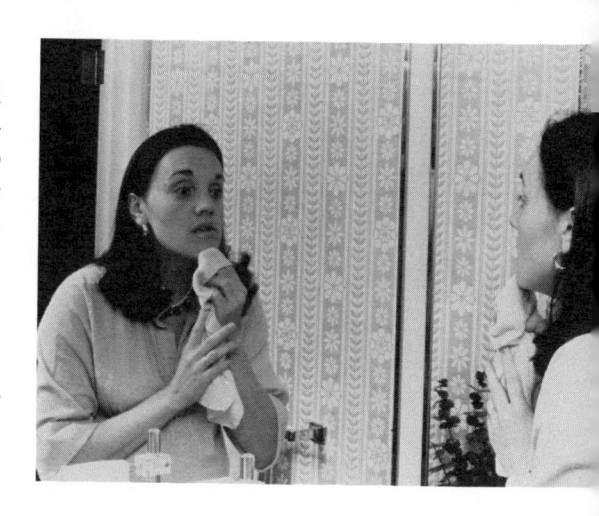

WHEN TO CALL YOUR DOCTOR

Usually, you feel quite good during postpartum, but sometimes variations from the normal postpartum pattern do occur. If you should experience any of the following, be sure to call your doctor:

- Excessive fatigue, despite adequate rest.
- Fever or chills.
- Abdominal cramps or tenderness. Afterpains are usually over by the time you go home.
- Bleeding that persists at home, becomes excessive, is bright red, or has a foul smell.
- Tenderness or redness in the calves of your legs.
- Sore, warm, or inflamed areas in your breasts; or red, cracked or bleeding nipples, which may signal mastitis.
- Burning sensations when you urinate, or frequent urges to urinate, which may signal a bladder infection.
- Severe or prolonged blues or depression.

NUTRITION

Calories

Nonpregnant women of childbearing age need approximately 2,100 calories a day to provide enough energy for good health and ordinary activity. During pregnancy you needed to increase your daily caloric intake to about 2,400 calories. If you are a breast-feeding mother you not only need to increase your daily caloric intake to about 2,700 calories, but you have to make every calorie count by planning a diet based on nutrient-rich foods.

Although the caloric or energy-producing needs of the breast-feeding mother increase by only about 30 percent (or 600 calories a day), the nutritional needs increase by as much as 60 percent. Your intake of protein is more important than your caloric intake when you are breast-feeding, and your needs for calcium, phosphorous, Vitamin A, and Vitamin C are all increased.

If you are bottle-feeding, you need a high-energy, well-balanced, low-calorie diet.

Nutrient Density

Some foods have a high nutrient density—they provide a maximum of nutrients with a minimum of calories. Foods in the "basic four" food groups are of this type. Foods of low-nutrient density provide a minimum of nutrients with a maximum of calories. These are the "junk foods"—candy, cake, pie, doughnuts, pastry, potato chips, pretzels, fried foods, and soda pop. Poor nutrition comes from not eating enough foods with high nutrient density. Make every calorie count.

Weight Loss

If you are overweight at the beginning of your postpartum period, be sure to cut back on high-calorie foods, empty of nutrients, rather than eliminating food high in protein, calcium, and vitamins. Postpartum is not the time to try to lose weight. You need all of the energy and vitality that a well-balanced diet can supply.

Nutrient-rich calorie-saving foods are skim milk, cottage cheese, plain yogurt, fresh fruits and vegetables, lean fish, and chicken.

Breast-feeding Mothers

If you are breast-feeding you can usually meet your added nutritional requirements by increasing slightly the amounts of milk, cheese, eggs, whole-wheat bread, and citrus juices in your diet. Since lactation itself burns a great number of calories, many women lose weight while breast-feeding.

Basic Food Groups

Whether you are bottle- or breast-feeding you and your family need a good diet that includes a variety of food from the four basic food groups: proteins, dairy products, cereals, and fruits and vegetables.

PROTEIN

When providing protein for your family, you have two choices: animal and vegetable. Animal proteins are considered "complete" since they contain the essential amino acids that your body needs to build and repair tissues. Sources of animal protein are meats, fish, poultry, eggs, milk, and cheese.

Vegetable proteins are called "incomplete" because they must be combined with one another to be used by your body. Good sources of vegetable protein are dried beans or peas, lentils, nuts and nut butters, sunflower seeds, and tofu (soybean curd).

If you are not breast-feeding, three servings, or six ounces, of protein are sufficient to meet your daily needs. However, if you are breast-feeding you must increase your daily intake to four servings or eight ounces of animal protein or an equivalent. One serving of two ounces of lean cooked meat supplies the same amount of protein as two eggs, one-half cup of cottage cheese, two slices of cheese, four tablespoons of peanut butter, or three-fourths of a cup of dried beans, peas, or lentils.

DAIRY PRODUCTS

Dairy products, which contain calcium, protein, fats, vitamins, and minerals, not only provide the nutrients you need to maintain and build tissues but also give you energy and help your body operate at peak efficiency. Milk and milk products help keep your skin glowing and healthy. The calcium in milk products improves your body's utilization of iron and assists in blood clotting.

When you are not breast-feeding, two cups of milk each day meet your nutritional needs. However, when you are breast-feeding, your requirements double and your milk intake should increase to four glasses a day. This can be taken in many forms. The calcium in one eight-ounce glass of whole or skim milk or buttermilk is equivalent to that found in one cup of yogurt, custard, or milk pudding, or in 1⅓ cups of cottage cheese or 1½ ounces of cheddar cheese.

CEREAL PRODUCTS

Cereals and whole grain products help supply you with carbohydrates that can be converted into a quick and efficient source of energy. They add fiber and bulk to your diet. Those rich in the B-complex vitamins aid in the proper functioning of your heart and nervous system and are important for healthy gums, teeth, and blood vessels. Iron-enriched products help to make hemoglobin, the red substance in your blood that carries oxygen to your cells.

Four servings of a whole-grain product fill your daily nutritional needs. One slice of whole-wheat or enriched bread is equal to one-half cup of brown rice, whole-grain macaroni, pasta, or grits. Two corn tortillas, one muffin, dumpling, pancake or waffle, or a two-inch square of cornbread are all equivalent to one bread or whole-grain serving.

FRUITS AND VEGETABLES

Fruits and vegetables provide you with important vitamins, minerals and fiber. By eating a variety of fruits and vegetables you receive all the necessary nutrients.

In your daily menu plans, include two servings each of vegetables and fruits to provide the proper amounts of vitamins A and C. Increase your usual intake of fruits, vegetables, and other high-fiber foods to help prevent constipation.

Vitamin A. Dark green vegetables such as spinach, broccoli, mustard greens, Brussels sprouts, kale, and cabbage supply you and your baby with Vitamin A, as well as other vitamins, iron, and magnesium. Yellow vegetables and fruits such as carrots, pumpkins, sweet potatoes, yams, apricots, and peaches help provide Vitamin A too.

Vitamin C. To obtain all the recommended daily requirements of Vitamin C and over half the Vitamin A necessary, include any of the following foods in your diet: one medium orange or ¾ cup (six ounces) of juice; ½ grapefruit or ¾ cup (six ounces) of juice; two medium tomatoes or two cups of juice; ½ large cantaloupe; one cup strawberries; ¾ cup broccoli; or 1½ cups cabbage.

Fluids

If you are brest-feeding, be sure to drink plenty of fluids, ten to twelve glasses a day. This ensures proper functioning of the bladder and bowels and helps build up your milk supply. One way to be sure you are getting adequate fluids is to drink a large glass of liquid each time you feed your baby.

REST AND SLEEP

Rest and sleep are times of restoration and are essential to your health. For a healthy, happy postpartum, it is vital to avoid becoming excessively tired. Although different women need different amounts of sleep, you should have enough rest to prevent your ending the day exhausted and irritable.

Sleep

To ensure good sleep, get exercise and fresh air during the day. Don't drink colas or coffee, which are high in caffeine, near bedtime. Before you go to bed, take a walk, have a warm bath, drink a glass of warm milk, or ask your husband to give you a massage.

Napping

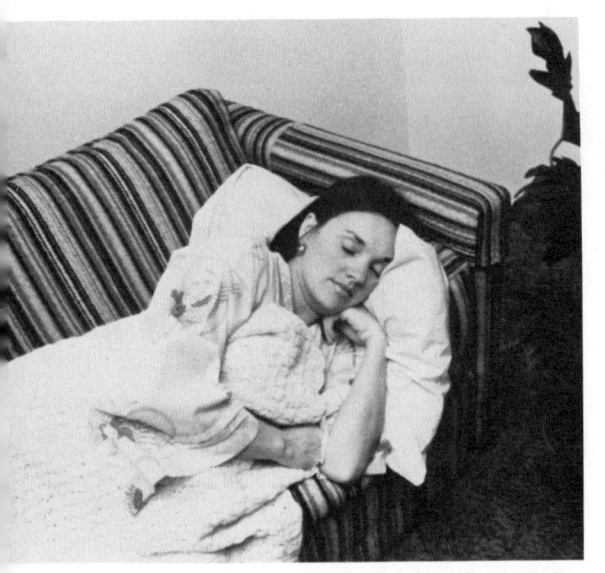

Whenever you feel tired during the day, take a nap. Napping is a very useful skill. Try to establish a daily pattern. Pull the blinds, take the phone off the hook, get out of your clothes, crawl into bed, cover yourself with blankets, close your eyes, and relax. Try napping when your baby naps. If you are breast-feeding, lay your baby next to you and breast-feed lying down.

Restricting Daily Activities

During the first day at home the new parents should be alone so they can settle in with their baby. Limit visitors the first week to close friends and those who will bring food and help you. Stay in your nightclothes this first week to remind yourself and others that you need rest. Try to alternate each hour of activity with an hour of resting with your feet up. Don't climb stairs if possible, and if you have stairs, don't climb them more than necessary. Don't lift heavy loads. Accept help from any and every source.

RELAXATION

Knowing the art of relaxation will benefit you for the rest of your life. Relaxation can help prevent the tension that makes you nervous, fatigued, and irritable. Relaxation does not mean sleep, but the ability to rest and relieve emotional strain. When you are tense it is hard to organize your life and set priorities.

Relaxation is a skill that needs to be practiced just as exercise does. Recognize situations, people, and places that cause you to become tense. Recognize situations that help you relax: warm baths, soothing music, a rocking chair, massage, perhaps a glass of warm beverage or wine. Try to avoid situations that make you tense; learn to choose situations that help you relax.

Slow, deep, comfortable breathing helps your blood circulation, and the soothing rhythm will help you relax. Learn to breathe correctly, with concentration and control. Take in a deep breath through your nose to warm and filter the air coming into the lungs. Then exhale through your pursed lips. Concentrate on what you are doing. Practice this when you rest or relax.

To practice relaxation exercises, find a comfortable position sitting or lying down. Take in a deep breath and tense your whole body. Exhale and relax your whole body.

Concentrate on feeling both the tension and the relaxation. Now, tense muscles in different parts of your body, and at the same time concentrate on making the rest of your body relax. When you feel in control of all the muscles in your body, take five more breaths and, with each breath, concentrate on relaxing even further. Think about being on a beach with warm sand, refreshing breeze, puffy clouds, and the sound of the surf. With each breath, feel your body slipping into the sand and becoming more and more relaxed. Each time you practice, try to get your body more relaxed than it has ever been before. Enjoy your session daily.

EXERCISE

The responsibilities of your new baby are sometimes so demanding that you may forget to get out and exercise. Exercise will make you feel better and react more efficiently. Weather permitting, try to get out for a brisk walk at least once a day. Fresh air and sunshine help to revitalize your spirits and give you a fresh perspective on life.

FATIGUE: PREVENTION

Probably the most common feeling you will have during your first weeks of mothering is fatigue. Changing, feeding, bathing your new baby, along with cooking and your customary household chores, may easily wear you out. Not only have you just emerged from the rigorous experience of childbirth, but you have the 24-hour-a-day charge of your newborn. That may mean feeding schedules every 2–3 hours day and night. Trying to take on too much too soon can leave you completely exhausted and depressed.

During the first weeks of motherhood you should be realistic about what you can accomplish. Get help with your housework. Hire baby-sitters and make sure you have plenty of rest. Don't expect to be superwoman. Allow yourself time to rest and recuperate. Don't expect to return to your nonpregnant state immediately after the birth of your baby. It takes at least six weeks for your body to recover and resume its former size and shape.

Don't try to be the perfect homemaker with a spotless house and elegant meals served exactly on time. Set a priority list for the most important tasks to be done in your house, then strike out all but the top five and let the rest go—not forever, just for a short time.

Don't expect to be the perfect wife. Your immediate concern is recuperation, and the 24-hour-a-day task of getting nourishment and care to your newborn. You cannot at the same time meet all your husband's needs. Sit down and discuss what you both can realistically expect from one another, and most important of all, recognize that this is just a very short time.

You cannot be a perfect mother, because you did not get a perfectly regulated baby. Your baby is unpredictable and needs time to mature in her habits and patterns. Do the best you can and do not let yourself feel guilty. In the next six weeks your baby will mature, and both you and she will develop more regular and predicatable schedules. Remember, being a mother is a learned task, so look for help from doctors, nurses, midwives, friends, relatives, clubs, and books. Use the information that fits your style and needs, and forget the rest.

Household Help

- Plan ahead for help in the house. If you can afford it, hire a part-time housekeeper.
- Call on your relatives, who may enjoy being with you and helping you at this time.
- Have lists made out of chores around the house. If friends ask what they can do to help you, point to the list of tasks. Friends enjoy helping.
- Call your nearby high school or college to see if they have students who are interested in helping new mothers with housekeeping chores or supervising your other children.

Meal Planning

- Before your baby is born, plan a couple of weeks' menus and make and freeze them for later use. Or, before your baby is born, cook double meals for two weeks, freezing one set.

- Take advantage of prepackaged convenience foods and stock up on them before your baby is born.
- Check restaurants in your area that have carry-out dinners and will deliver them.
- If your friends or relatives want to give you a baby shower suggest one in which they bring meals that you can put in your freezer, or have them arrange delivery of one meal each evening for two weeks.
- If your husband enjoys cooking, stock the refrigerator with ingredients he requests and let him develop his gourmet skills.
- Friends appreciate being needed. When they ask what they can do, mention how much a meal would be appreciated.

Childcare

- If your mother or mother-in-law wants to give you a gift, ask for a month's diaper service in which your baby's dirty diapers are picked up and clean ones left.
- Call your visiting nurse service. The nurse can help answer any questions you have about your newborn. She may also assess your needs for a homemaker's service.
- If you are bottle-feeding you may try to use prepared formula for the first couple of weeks to cut down on your work.
- Use disposable diapers the first couple of weeks.
- Encourage your husband to share baby care. He will learn about and enjoy his baby faster when he is involved with bathing, feeding, and nurturing her. Don't criticize the way he holds, changes, or bathes the baby, but allow him to do it his way.
- Stay in bed to nurse and nap while you are feeding your baby. If night feedings are exhausting, have your husband bring the baby to you.

11.

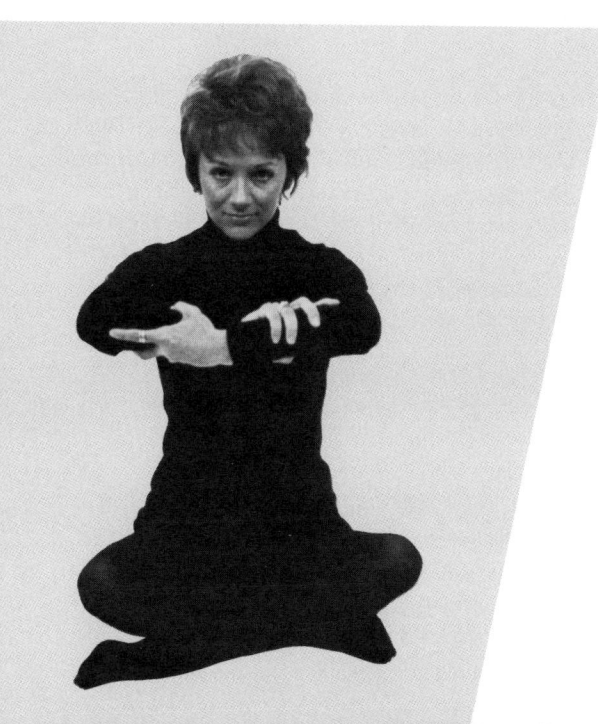

Postnatal Exercises

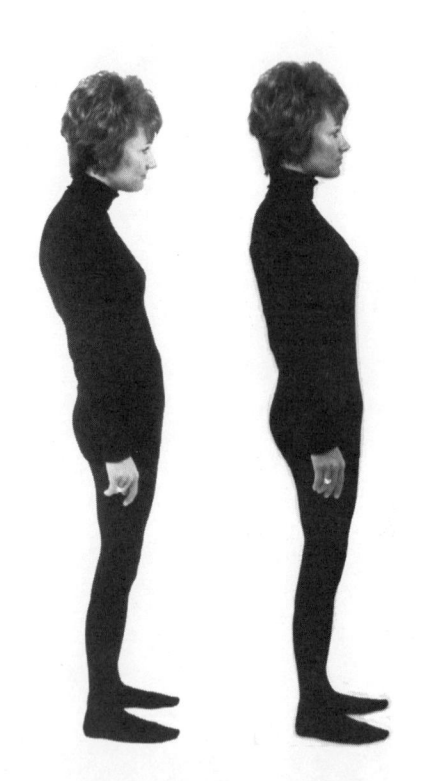

Like most women you are probably anxious to lose the weight you gained during pregnancy. You may be concerned by the sight of your flabby abdominal muscles. Although full recovery takes at least six weeks, if you exercise every day, you can begin to regain your strength and your figure.

Postnatal exercises are designed to help strengthen the muscles that were stretched during pregnancy, labor, and delivery. The exercises are divided into two sets: those you may begin the first six weeks after delivery, and the more rigorous ones designed for the following six-week period.

When you arrive home your uterus is about twice the size it was before pregnancy. Within the next six weeks, as it shrinks to normal size, overactivity or activity resumed too early will slow this crucial process. In the first weeks after birth there are dangers of delayed hemorrhage or of infection.

You may begin the first nine exercises on the first day following delivery, then add the others on the third or fourth day. At first do each exercise 3–5 times, twice a day, and work up to 10 times each at least twice a day. Be careful not to exercise too much too soon. The color and flow of your vaginal discharge are good indications of whether or not you are overdoing. If the flow increases or becomes bright red, stop exercising; then gradually resume activity.

During the first week, exercise gently and never to the point of discomfort. The pelvic floor exercise, the head lift, and the pelvic tilt are recommended for the first week.

FIRST SIX WEEKS

Posture

Poor posture causes backaches and makes you look slouchy and swaybacked. The added weight of pregnancy often emphasizes the problem.

To stand correctly, tuck in your buttocks, tilt your pelvis forward to align or straighten your spine, pull your shoulders back, arms relaxed, and hold your head erect with your chin in. Practice good posture and make it a habit for the rest of your life.

Pelvic Floor Exercise

The birth of a baby can stretch the muscles surrounding your vagina. This may affect the support of the reproductive organs and make it difficult to control urination. Strengthening these muscles will also enhance sexual pleasure for you and your partner.

You can practice the pelvic floor exercise while standing, sitting, or lying down. First, think of the openings on the pelvic floor. Push as if you were urinating and then pull up and in as if to stop the flow. Hold for a second, slowly release the tension, and repeat. If it is difficult to get the feeling of this exercise, do it when you are actually urinating. Gently, yet firmly and slowly, stop the flow several times and hold. This will make you aware of the action of these muscles.

Because it is important to perform this pelvic floor exercise regularly and often, practice it every time you do some commonplace activity, such as opening the refrigerator or looking in the mirror. Practice this exercise every time you make love.

Head Lift

The head lift helps to strengthen the abdominal muscles. Lie on your back on the floor, tilting your pelvis forward. Slowly inhale through your nose. Then slowly exhale through pursed lips as you draw your abdomen in and down as hard as possible, raising your head up off the floor throughout the exhalation.

Pelvic Tilt

The pelvic tilt will strengthen the abdominal muscles and stretch the lower back. Lie on your back with your knees bent and feet flat on the floor. Inhale through your nose and press the small of your back firmly against the floor by tightening your abdominal muscles and squeezing your buttocks together. The upper pelvis, your hips, will tilt back and down toward the floor. Hold this position while slowly exhaling through pursed lips; then relax and inhale.

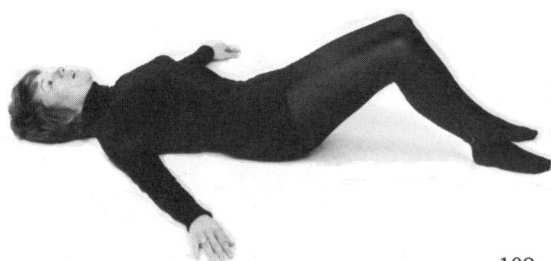

Elbow Circles

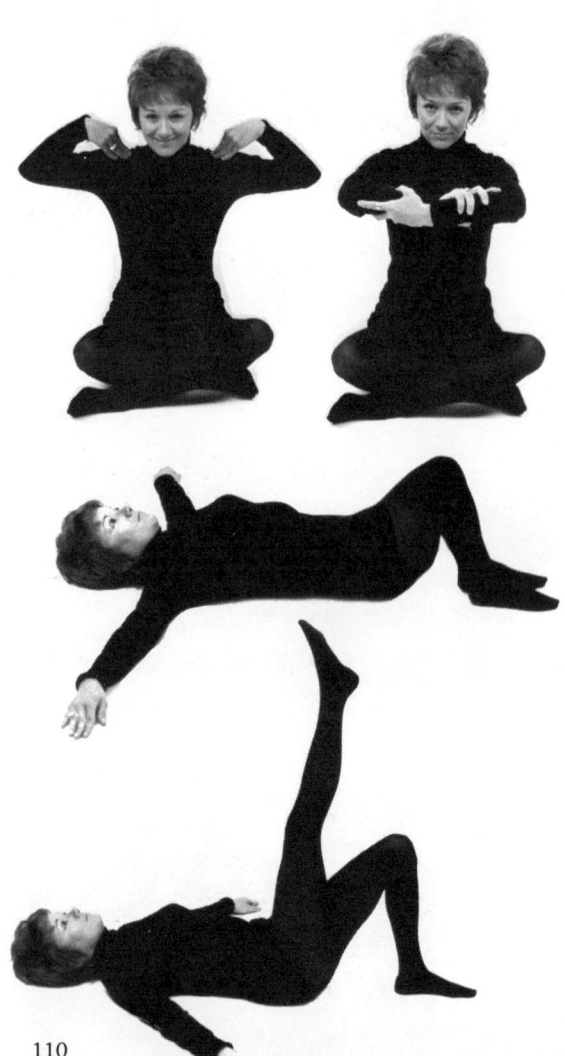

Elbow circles help to increase circulation in your chest area. Sitting with your fingertips on your shoulders, bring your elbows together, in front of you. Then move them up, around, out to the side, then down.

Elbow Press

To increase circulation in your breasts and keep them firm, do the elbow press. Raise your arms to shoulder height, bend your elbows, and put your palms together. Press and hold for a count of four. Release slowly and press again. You can get the same result by grasping each wrist with the opposite hand and, holding tightly, pushing to tense the muscles.

Knee Roll

The knee roll strengthens the oblique or diagonal muscles of your abdomen. Lie on your back with knees bent, arms out. With your feet flat on the floor, roll your knees to the right, keeping your shoulders flat at all times. Return to the starting position and roll your knees to the left. As strength increases, do this with your feet up off the floor.

Leg Lift

The leg lift is another exercise that strengthens the abdominal muscles and improves circulation in your legs. Lie on your back with legs bent. Tilt your pelvis forward. Slowly lift one leg as high as possible while inhaling through your nose; then slowly lower your leg while exhaling through pursed lips. Switch leg positions and lift your other leg.

Pelvic Lift

The pelvic lift strengthens the buttocks and backs of the thighs and stretches the fronts of the thighs. Lie on your back with knees bent, feet flat on the floor. Lift your pelvis up, but do not arch your back. Squeeze your knees and buttocks together and inhale through your nose. Slowly lower your pelvis back to the floor while exhaling through pursed lips.

Partial Sit-up

Partial sit-ups also help strengthen your abdominal muscles. Lying on your back with knees bent, feet flat on the floor, tilt your pelvis forward with your back flat against the floor. Raise your head and shoulders, attempting to roll up to a sitting position. Hold for a slow count of five, and then slowly uncurl and relax.

SECOND SIX WEEKS

After six-weeks you should have the strength and energy to do more strenuous exercises, which are effective in getting rid of tummy bulge, firming up your buttocks and thighs, and losing any excess fatty deposits. The exercises put special emphasis on the abdominal muscles, both the longitudinal (from the center front of the lower ribs to the pubic bone) and the oblique (stretching from the lower ribs in a wide diagonal sheet to the opposite hip).

All exercises should be done very slowly, since muscles have to work harder when no momentum is built up. Pick those exercises you need and enjoy, and exercise daily. Don't forget to keep up the pelvic floor exercise, which will benefit you for the rest of your life.

Hip Hiking

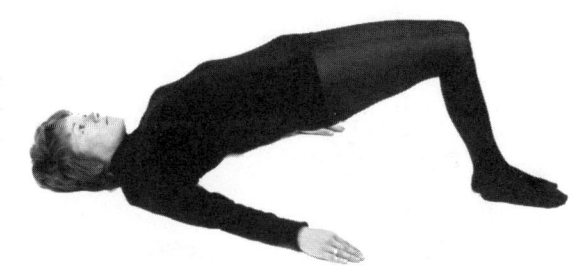

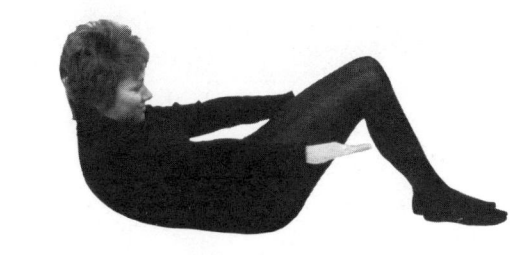

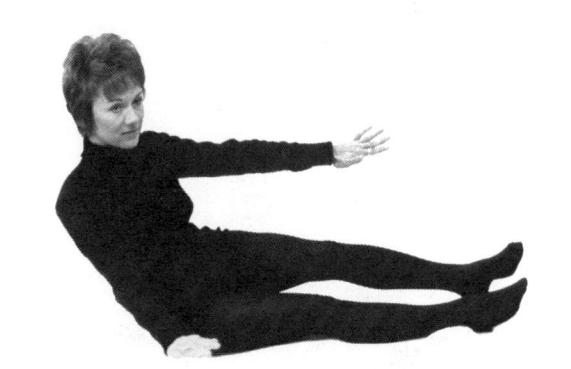

Hip hiking slims and tones up your waist and thighs. Sit with your legs straight out in front, and your arms out to the side. Lift your right hip and leg two to three inches off the floor. Repeat on the other side. Feel the lift coming from the muscles at the hip, the side of your waist, and the front of your thigh.

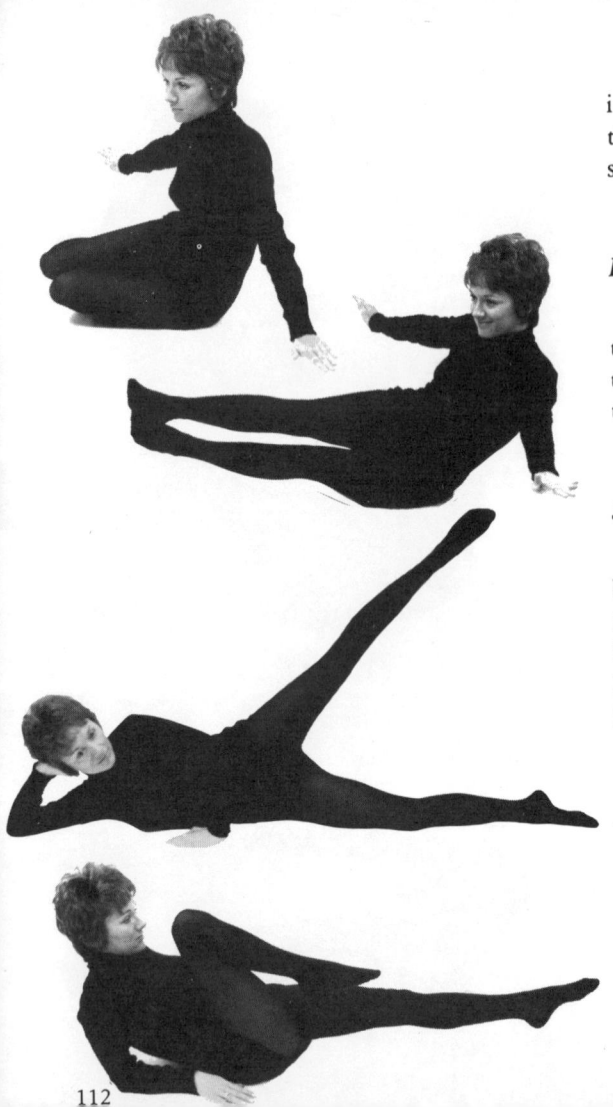

Kneel Sitting

Kneel sitting helps to strengthen your thighs, hips, and abdominal muscles. In a sitting position bend your knees to one side of your body. Stretch your legs forward without touching the floor while balancing on one hip, and bend your legs back again. Repeat on the other side.

Side Leg Raise

The side leg raise will strengthen and firm up your outer and inner thigh muscles and buttocks. Lie on your side with one hand propping up your head and the other on the floor in front of you balancing your body. Slowly raise your upper leg, holding it a little behind you. Do not let it come forward. Relax your foot; don't point your toes. Slowly lower your leg. Repeat several times. Using your arms for balance and bracing, raise both legs up, keeping knees and ankles squeezed tightly together. Repeat on the other side.

Horizontal Bicycle

The horizontal bicycle will strengthen the longitudinal abdominal muscles. Sit with your legs stretched out in front of you, propping yourself up on your elbows. Tilt your pelvis. Bring your right knee to your chest, and then lift your left leg up three inches off the floor. As in bicycling, reverse the motion by bringing the left knee to your chest and stretching out your right leg three inches above the floor. Repeat. Never have both legs stretched out above the floor at once, as it could cause lower back strain.

Side Bicycle

The side bicycle strengthens the oblique muscles of your abdomen. Lie on your back, arms out at each side, both knees bent up toward your chest, with your shoulders flat on the floor. Roll to the right; bicycle four circles, keeping the legs off the floor. Repeat on the other side.

Pelvic Raising

Pelvic raising strengthens muscles in your buttocks, lower back, and the backs of the thighs and abdomen. Lie on your back, legs straight, with feet up on a stool or low chair. Raise your pelvis as you inhale through the nose; lower your pelvis to the right side as you exhale. Raise it up again and lower it to the left side. Repeat.

Modified Sit-ups

Modified sit-ups help to strengthen your abdominal muscles, both longitudinal and oblique. Lie on your back, legs bent, with feet flat on the floor. Do a pelvic tilt, pressing the small of your back against the floor. Inhale. Reach forward and roll up to a sitting position. Exhale. Repeat, curling to the right, diagonally, and once more curling to the left.

Airplane

The airplane strengthens thighs and abdomen. Lie on your back, legs straight, arms out to each side. Raise one leg up and over to the opposite side, keeping the knees straight, and attempt to touch your toe to the opposite hand. Repeat with the opposite leg.

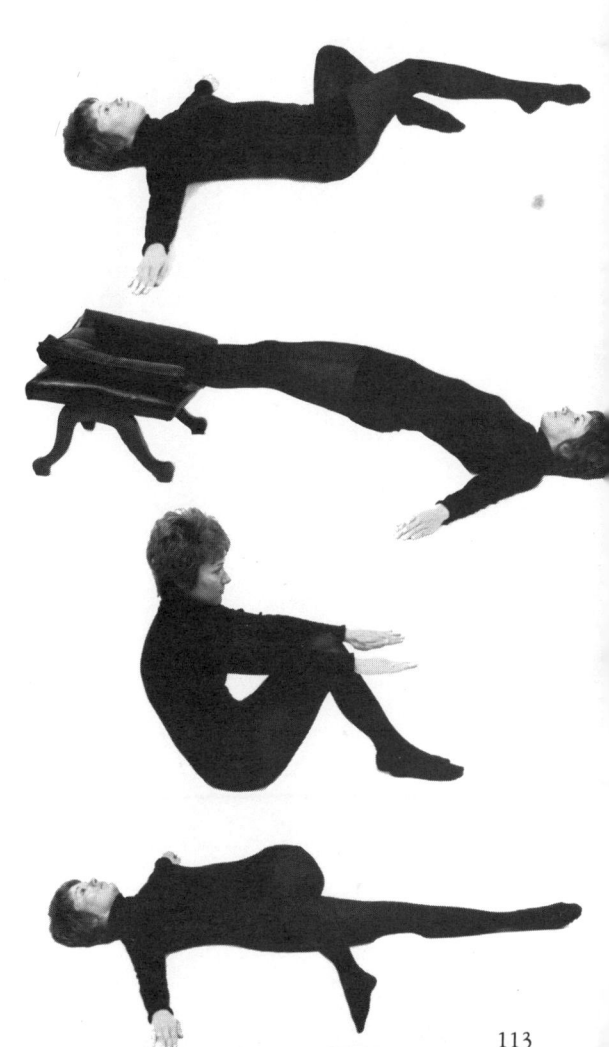

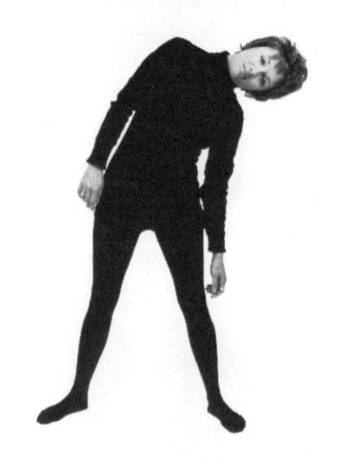

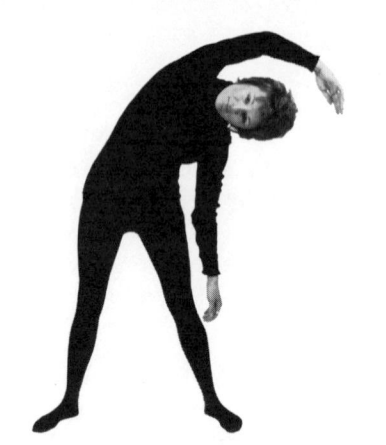

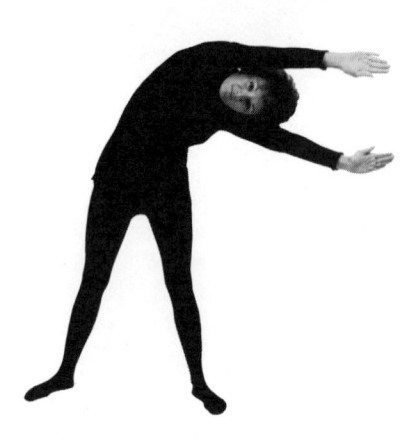

Side Bending

Use side bending to slim your waist. Stand with your feet well apart and bend to the right side three times, then three times to the left.

With your right arm over your head, bend to the right side three times. Repeat on the left.

With both arms over your head for added weight, bend to the right side three times. Don't lean forward. Repeat on the left side.

EXERCISE TIME

If you exercise every day for even fifteen minutes, you will notice improvements within two weeks. Of course, doing them twice a day is better yet, but even twice a week is better than not at all, and will make a difference.

There is a strong link between physical and mental health. Not only will exercise aid in maintaining good physical condition, but it also gives you a sense of well-being. Good health gives you the energy you need to enjoy your baby and your new life.

12.

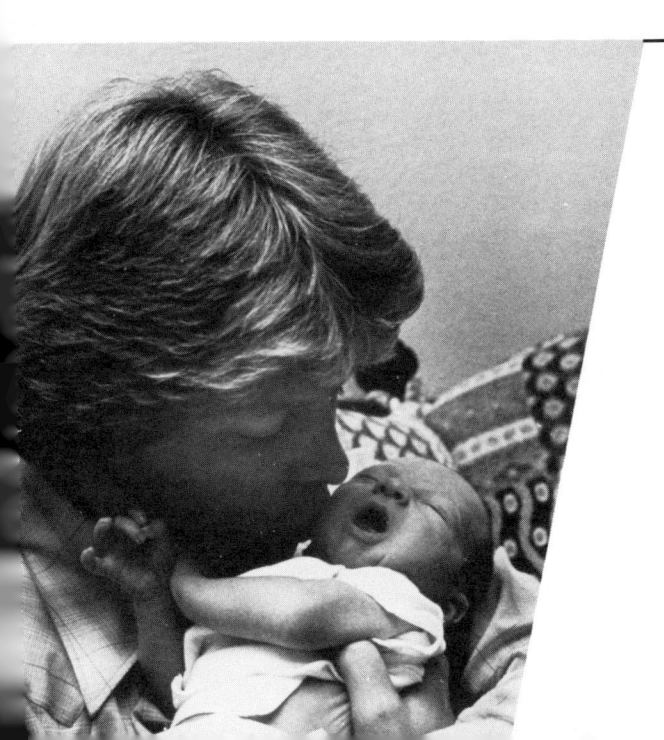

Changing Roles

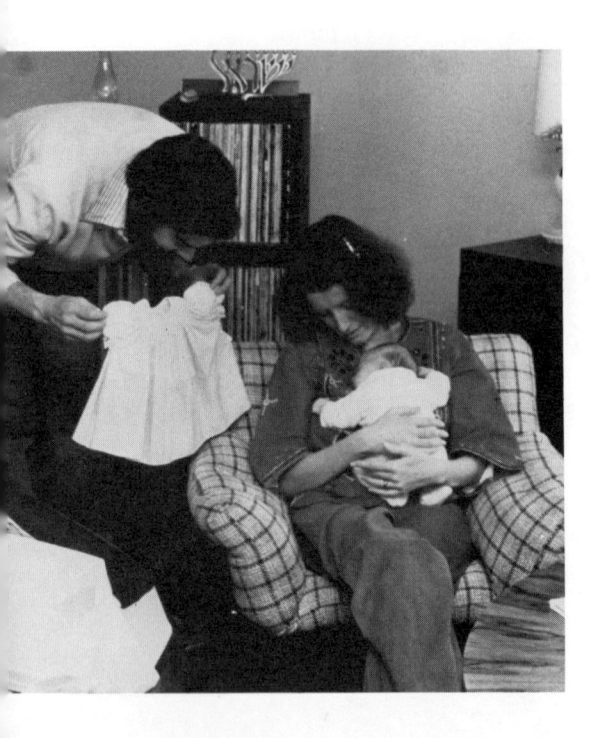

Fluctuating emotions are a normal response to the tremendous change the new baby brings to your family. It is natural for new parents to have a range of feelings from ecstasy to depression. The most common moods are joy, exhaustion, tension, and fatigue. Lack of confidence in your ability to nurture and soothe your baby is common.

When you bring your baby home, you may be surprised by the demands the newborn makes on your time, leaving you as a couple few moments to share together. Night feedings can leave both of you suffering from lack of sleep. You may be frustrated in your initial attempts to learn about your baby, especially in knowing what soothes and stimulates her.

Although early postpartum is a time of change and moments of frustration, it is also a time of joy and happiness. You, the mother and father, will feel that you are growing and maturing. Your concept of yourself will expand to include your role as a parent, and you will probably experience feelings of satisfaction with this role. For many couples, the meaning of life and death is heightened. The following are some parents' thoughts during early postpartum:

- "I find myself growing and changing every day along with my baby."
- "I feel myself more whole as a person."
- "I feel as if I have created a miracle."
- "I listen to my baby's heartbeat and am overwhelmed by the significance of this human being who is the total creation of myself and my husband."
- "I appreciate the total cycle of life and death."

EMOTIONAL CHANGES—THE MOTHER

Lack of Confidence

Although parenthood is one of the most important tasks in life, it is one career for which few people are equipped with a college degree or trade apprenticeship. The newborn you give birth to comes to you with immature systems, unpredictable responses, and cues that you must learn to interpret and respond to. As she matures, your job becomes easier and easier. But during the first weeks you may be disappointed in your ability to cope and you may lack confidence. It helps if you recognize that your baby is a resilient being who can withstand many mistakes. After all, nature has equipped mothers with instincts that have worked for millions of years. Have faith in your own innate ability to mother and listen to your instincts about your baby. Be yourself, don't try to be a super mother. Choose friends and relatives whom you respect and ask for their advice. Choose a doctor who gives you confidence and don't hesitate to call him. Surround yourself with positive, confidence-building friends who have had babies. Renew your relationship with your own mother and let her share in your experience. If you have a fussy child, do all you can to console and comfort her and don't blame yourself for her crying. Leave the baby, even if you have to leave her with a baby-sitter, for half an hour; get out and take a walk.

Hostility

As a new mother you may experience feelings of hostility toward your baby because of the tremendous amount of work she has brought into your life and because of your feelings of inadequacy when you cannot comfort or console her. You may also feel hostile toward your husband, who is free to get dressed up, leave the house, go out to lunch, and come home at the end of the day. Recognize hostility as a normal feeling toward your baby, yourself, and your partner. Define and verbalize how you are feeling to your husband. Confide in a sympathetic friend who has recently experienced childbirth. Reexamine your priorities and find your own style that works for you, not what women's magazines think is right. Be realistic in your role. Motherhood and fatherhood are not always serene and calm, and there are many storms ahead. Listen to each other's feelings and concerns. Set realistic expectations for both of you. Try to search for workable alternatives. Don't make demands of one another, instead, try to communicate.

Poor Self-Esteem

All your new responsibilities in your career as a parent may lower your self-esteem. You don't look as good as you thought you would, your patience may be wanting, and you are seldom sure that what you're doing as a parent is right. Confide in a friend who has experienced parenthood and is sympathetic. Take time out for yourself alone. Outside activities, walking, and exercise classes will help you gain perspective. Read interesting books, get out to shop for a new outfit that you look good in. Have your hair done. Reexamine your expectations of yourself and set up realistic priorities. Ask your husband to share in the tasks of housekeeping and baby caretaking; it will help him develop sympathy and compassion. Go out to a candlelight dinner (if you are breast-feeding you can take the baby with you), or to a movie.

Confinement

Having 24-hour-a-day charge of a new baby can easily lead to feelings of confinement. It is important that you continue your life as a person and that you get out of the house to keep a perspective on life. Take your baby out with you. You can use a Snugli, carrier, or stroller. The fresh air is as good for her as it is for you. Leave your baby with her father and take a walk by yourself. Get a baby-sitter, and either go out by yourself or stay at home and enjoy yourself while your baby is being looked after. Join a baby-sitting co-op or leave your baby with a friend in whom you have faith. Take your baby with you to the park, movie, restaurant. You may not feel like taking part in community activities with your newborn, but as she matures plan to take time out for creative activities, adult education courses, recreation, and volunteer work. As your baby gets older, you may even find you enjoy your baby more if you leave her with a reliable baby-sitter and find some type of part-time work you find interesting. For those of you who plan to return to full-time work it is important that you keep in touch with your employer about your plans for returning.

Guilt

It is common for both the mother and father to feel guilty about their negative feelings toward their child and toward each other. The newborn takes a great deal of time that you could have spent together. When she cries you have to jump; and, if you have an irritable baby, this feeling of guilt is intensified. You may fear that your nonmaternal and nonpaternal feelings are abnormal. First, accept that these feelings are normal and okay. You may have unrealistic expectations about yourself as a parent and a partner. What women's magazines think a "good mother" should be, and what a good mother really is, can be two different things. In order to be a good mother, you must first feel good about yourself. Whether you plan to return to full-time employment or prefer to stay home and enjoy mothering, don't feel guilty about not being a supermom. Ask for help when you need it. Communicate your feelings to your husband (he probably has experienced the same feelings). Try to engage in activities that help you feel better about yourself.

Depression: The Blues

Although at the birth you may have felt the joyous emotions of new parenthood, soon thereafter you may experience what is called "postpartum blues." Postpartum depression is an overwhelming feeling that you are helpless and unable to cope with your baby. It can happen right after birth or, more usually, on the fourth or fifth day of postpartum; or, even a month after your baby is born. You may cry for no apparent reason or feel insecure about handling your baby. You may feel estranged from your husband and believe that your baby has ended your freedom to live your life as you wish. These "blues" are experienced by about 60 percent of all women sometime during the first ten days following birth.

Depression is a common occurrence in the first days of motherhood. Along with fatigue and exhaustion, you may be experiencing physical discomfort from your stitches and from coping with a heavy vaginal flow. Your milk may have just come in and you may suffer from engorgement and sore nipples.

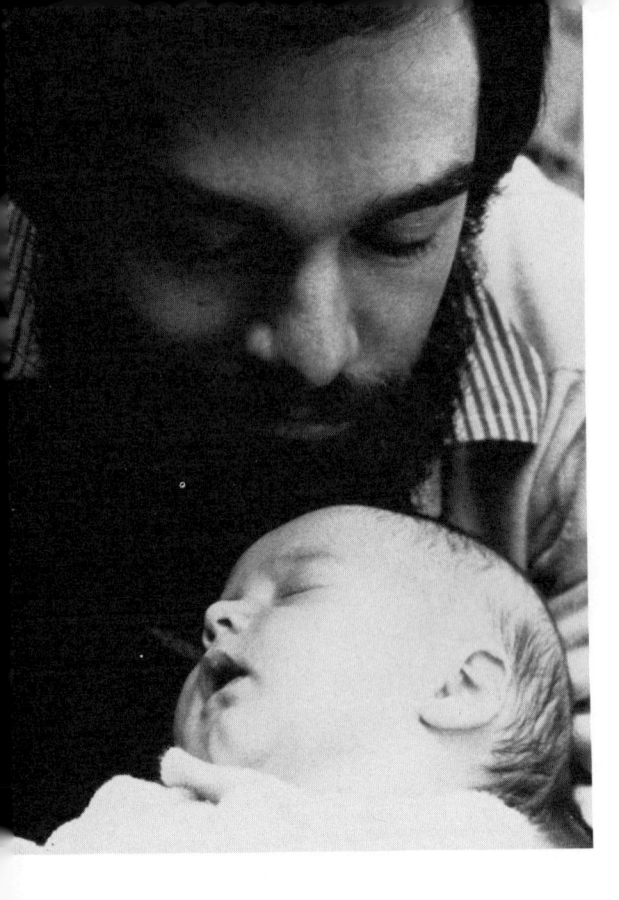

Another cause of depression is the dramatic hormonal changes that take place in your body following birth. When the placenta is delivered, the amount of estrogen and progesterone drops suddenly and this alone can trigger depression.

Although the exact causes of most postpartum depression are not known, it would be safe to say that fatigue plays a great part. Try to keep yourself from becoming overwhelmingly exhausted. However, if you do become depressed, realize that it is a natural and common part of postpartum and will soon fade away. It is helpful to talk to friends who have experienced it. Fathers and even adoptive parents can experience postpartum blues.

Some feelings of depression are almost certain to occur in varying degrees sometime during your six-week postpartum period. If possible, your mother, a relative, or a friend should be available to help you during the first few weeks following birth. Round-the-clock baby tending can be physically and psychologically fatiguing. Rest, with breaks from childcare and household duties, can help prevent physical and mental exhaustion.

The common "postpartum blues" are episodes of fluctuating and short-lived tearful periods. On the other hand, serious postpartum depression (experienced by 10 percent of women) is identified by an intense and long-lasting mood change that impairs a woman's ability to function.

If your depression does not subside but instead leaves you incapable of assuming your normal responsibilities and activities, talk to your doctor or medical caregiver, who can give you the kind of help and support you need.

EMOTIONAL CHANGES—THE FATHER

You will probably feel great pride and joy toward the baby that you both created, especially if you were an active participant in the labor and delivery of your baby. You may be engrossed with your child, holding, cuddling, exploring, and taking photographs to capture the precious early hours and days of life. You will probably feel tender and protective toward your wife. Together you will want to relive the birth, moment by moment.

Let-down

After the birth, if your baby was delivered in a traditional hospital delivery room, you may feel quite let down. The great event of birth that you have looked forward to for so long is over and you were left outside and alone. It is important that you look to others for support at this time.

Overwhelmed

When your baby and wife come home from the hospital you may become overwhelmed by the reality of fatherhood. You may be awed by the impact of 24-hour-a-day, 7-days-a-week, 52-weeks-a-year responsibility for the next 20 years.

Hostility and Jealousy

While feeling tender and protective toward your wife and baby, you may be jealous of all the attention showered on them. Your life has turned upside down. Your ambivalent emotions may confuse and depress you. At the same time, the mother is also feeling ambivalent, and you may both wonder if you are ready for all this.

Fatigue and Exhaustion

Fatigue and exhaustion, from caring for the baby and night feedings, may intensify everything that you are feeling.

Anxiety and Depression

It is not uncommon for young fathers to feel trapped and to experience anxiety over finances and the future. You may be concerned about the imbalance between your own sex drive and the diminished sex drive of your wife. Some fathers even experience the postpartum blues following the birth of their baby.

Appreciation and Compassion

Some fathers choose to stay home to share in household tasks and help care for their wives and babies during the early week or weeks of life. Men who do this experience a sense of compassion toward their wives and a heightened appreciation of the specialness of their baby. This bonding seems an important part of the family experience. Although some fathers do not wish to share in the care of their infants, it is valuable for the father not to miss the joy of seeing his baby develop and grow. But the success of the father-child relationship depends a great deal upon the mother's willingness to give the father a chance to become involved with his baby. This may be a common response for some men. She should make sure that he takes part in feeding, soothing, playing, and nurturing their baby and thus build that sense of family that is so valuable.

Both boys and girls need a strong relationship with their father as well as with their mother. As your baby grows, he or she identifies with each parent and uses both parents as models to develop his or her sense of individuality. Your child needs both of you for as long as possible.

SUPPORT FOR THE MOTHER

Every new mother needs special protection, love, attention, and ego building. Marriage was never meant to provide it all. To help you through the first weeks of parenting, surround yourself with people who make you feel good about yourself as a person, and on whom you can rely.

Yourself

You bring with you to motherhood a reservoir of strength and resources. The qualities of tenderness, patience, enthusiasm, humor, compassion, empathy, sympathy, responsiveness, adaptability, flexibility, resiliency, endurance, versatility, tolerance, persistence, determination, perseverance, and faith will all be important in your parenting experience. Be confident that you have the natural instincts to do the right thing at the right time.

Your Partner

Your partner is one of your most important supports. Don't be afraid to disclose your feelings to him and discuss your needs. Learn to define what the real and important problems are. Brainstorm solutions together. Discuss their consequences and come to mutually acceptable solutions.

Your Family

Birth is a time for opening new avenues of communication with your family. The extended family can provide valuable emotional support during your pregnancy, birth, and in the early weeks of being a parent. Your relationship with your mother, who has just experienced becoming a grandmother, can become deeper and richer. She is probably reliving your birth and her parenting of you. If you look back with positive feelings about the mothering you received, it is not uncommon for you to develop a closer relationship with her. If you do not have positive feelings about some aspects of her parenting, you may consciously resolve to change those patterns and be a different kind of mother.

Your Friends

Having a friend who has recently experienced childbirth is an important source of support. There is no one who is more sympathetic or willing to share in your needs and concerns and to offer help. However, it is important to remember that each individual's problems need individual solutions. Your friend's experiences may not fit you or your baby's personality and style.

Medical Caregivers

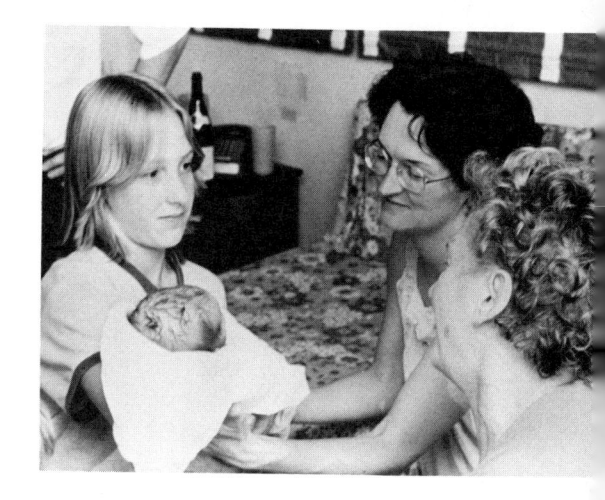

Pick a doctor in whom you have confidence and who respects you as an individual and gives you confidence in yourself. After the birth of your baby you may be confronted with a whole new series of problems: those that deal with you and your changing body and those that deal with your newborn and her body's immature systems. You will need a great deal of support and information from both the doctor or medical caregiver who accompanied you during your pregnancy and childbirth and also the person whom you have chosen to help guide you through your early mothering experience. Whether this person is the same (such as a general practitioner or family practitioner) or two specialists (such as an obstetrician and a pediatrician), it is extremely important that you can turn to a person in whom you have confidence and whom you can count on to give you help when you need it.

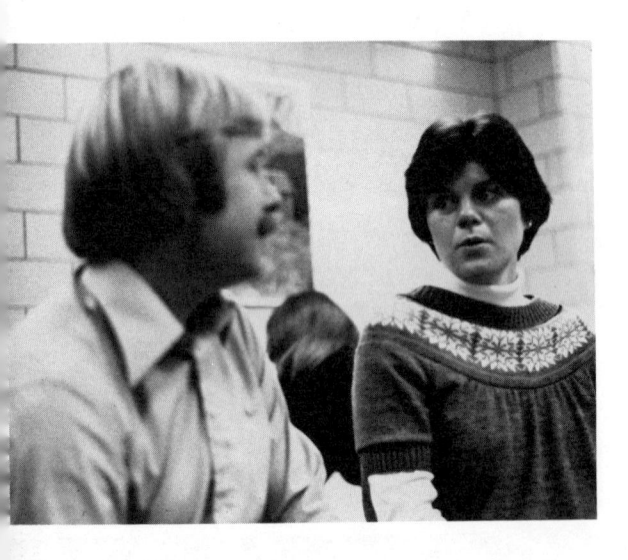

Parenting Classes

Groups of new mothers can give support and information to each other. Such groups are sponsored by hospitals, YWCAs, the Red Cross, and other organizations. An invaluable group who support breast-feeding mothers, called La Leche League, has helped many women successfully breast-feed their babies.

Community

Neighbors, churches, schools, adult education groups—all are there to help you in your parenting task. Remember, parenting was never supposed to be a lonely task. Throughout the history of mankind it has been shared by all members of the family and the community. It is your right and your responsibility to find support to help you enjoy parenting.

Other Sources

Bookstores and libraries abound with "how to" literature on parenting. There are voluminous amounts of information available. However, remember to use only the information that you feel comfortable with. There is no right way, only the one that helps you enjoy parenting your newborn.

SUPPORT FOR THE FATHER

It is as important for you, the father, to develop support groups as it is for the mother. Just because you are now a parent doesn't mean that you no longer need parenting. You will probably never need support more than you need it now.

Yourself

As a man, you are undergoing changes in roles as a person, husband, and father. You may still be in the process of adjusting to being a husband. As you try to adjust to your new role as a father, you will often think of your own father and how he parented you. You bring with you to the role of fatherhood your strengths of patience, adaptability, self-esteem, flexibility, tenderness, and compassion in varying degrees.

Your Partner

Although your partner may be overwhelmed and fatigued with the birth and the new baby, she brings to you her love and her needs. It is only for a short time in your lives that she will need you with such intensity. If you can meet some of her needs, you will develop qualities in your marriage that will strengthen it immeasurably.

Your Family

It is especially important that, if possible, you turn to your own family, especially your father and brothers, for their physical and emotional support. You may find your own father reliving his experience of your birth. Your mother may wish to help you handle the many household chores that she knows are involved with a new baby.

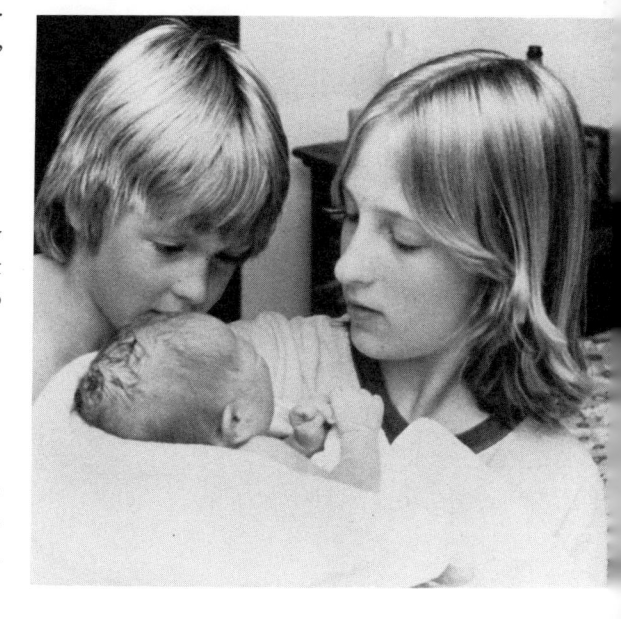

Your Friends

Surround yourself with friends who have recently experienced childbirth and parenting a newborn. They will share their experiences. Most important, they can help you gain the perspective that this is a temporary period that will pass.

Other Sources

You, as well as the mother, can look to your community for support. Parenting classes, churches, schools, and adult education groups may offer you support in terms of information and confidence. It may help you to read the many books that tell you about parenting and the newborn.

13.

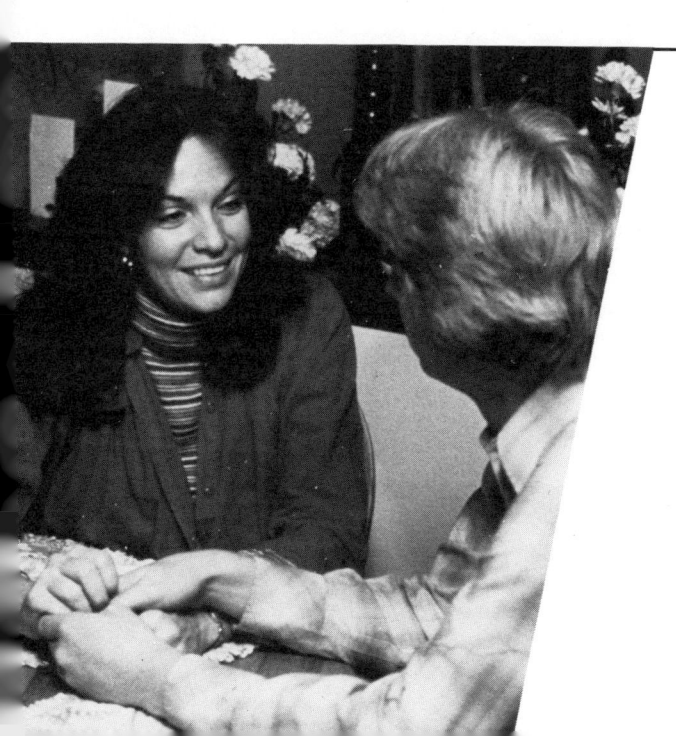

Your Marriage

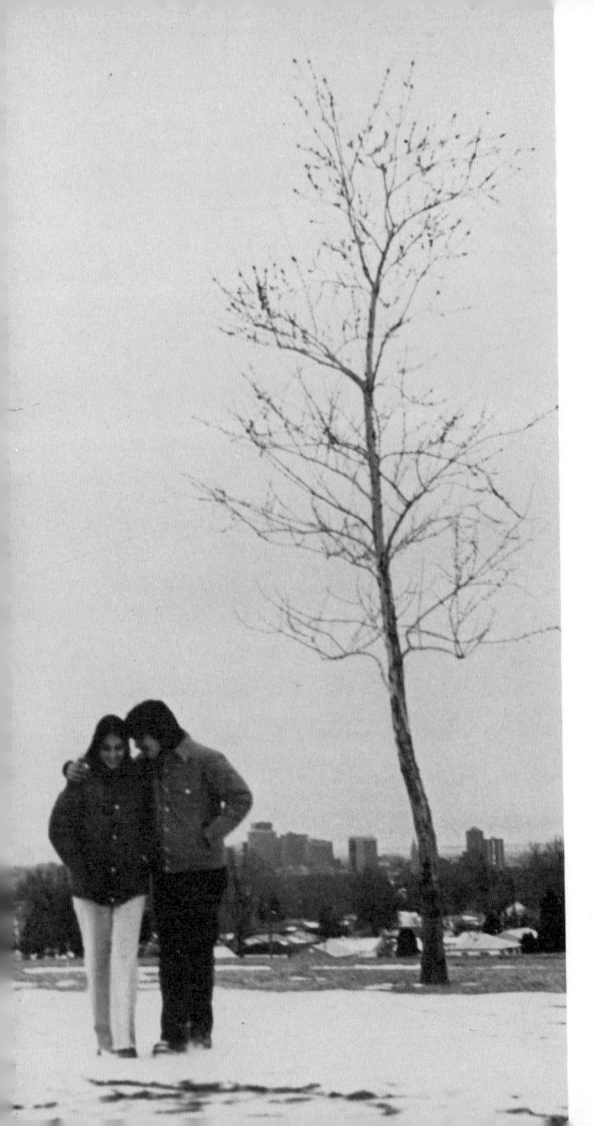

Your marriage's success depends a great deal on how both of you face and cope with stressful situations. If parenthood occurs before you have come to grips with the stresses of marriage, the stability of your relationship may be severely threatened. On the other hand, the shared act of conception and pregnancy can strengthen your marriage and deepen your relationship.

Pregnancy and childbirth are probably one of the first major crises that a young couple face together. The patterns of coping that you establish at this time will probably be followed in dealing with other life crises. Most marriages are deeply affected by the birth of a baby:

- "We have a new appreciation of the system of life as we see our baby change every day."
- "We have, through our child, reached out to other human beings and have greater empathy for others."
- "We are more realistic in our overview of life and have more general social awareness."
- "It has made us closer, more inseparable and dependent on each other."
- "I appreciate my husband's consideration and help as never before."
- "We have a greater appreciation of each other."
- "We share in the delight of fulfilling the needs of our baby."
- "I know now what they mean when they say, 'You are not really married until you have a baby.'"

At the same time, it is not unusual for a new baby to act as a wedge in your relationship and drive you apart. The 24-hour-a-day, 7-day-a-week care of your baby may overwhelm you. The combination of fatigue, a crying baby, fear of pregnancy, physical discomfort, lack of vaginal lubrication, and a diminished sex drive may result in an unsatisfactory sex life. You both may feel a need for more attention and support and yet have less time and energy to give it to one another. This is a time when communication and sensitivity to each other's needs are especially important.

HAVING FUN

It may be easy for the enjoyment of life to escape you during this period of your lives. Don't let this happen. You must make special efforts to do the things you enjoy together. Although there are some things you will have to give up temporarily because of your new baby, talk together about the things that gave you the greatest fun before the baby was born. Check off those that are impossible for six weeks and put them aside for another day. Decide which ones are possible—walking together, reading together, eating out, going to the movies, watching television, cooking, making fudge, popping popcorn, driving, concerts, swimming, visiting friends—and do them.

REDISCOVERING YOUR RELATIONSHIP

Reexplore your past and your marriage. How did you meet? What attracted you to one another? When did you know you were in love? When and why did you decide to get married? How did pregnancy change your marriage? How has this new baby enriched your relationship? Discuss the places where you have had the most fun together. Was it on your honeymoon, camping in the mountains, at the seashore, in a motel, in your own house, in your own bedroom? Which times do you remember that you were together that gave you joy? Your marriage, your birthday, anniversaries, when you found out you were pregnant, the birth of your baby?

Rediscover each other. Tell your partner those qualities that you love best in her. What do you like best about the way he looks? What special qualities does she have that you love? How is he different from others and why did you choose him? What does she do that you like best of all? When you are sad or depressed what does your partner do that helps you?

COMMUNICATION SKILLS

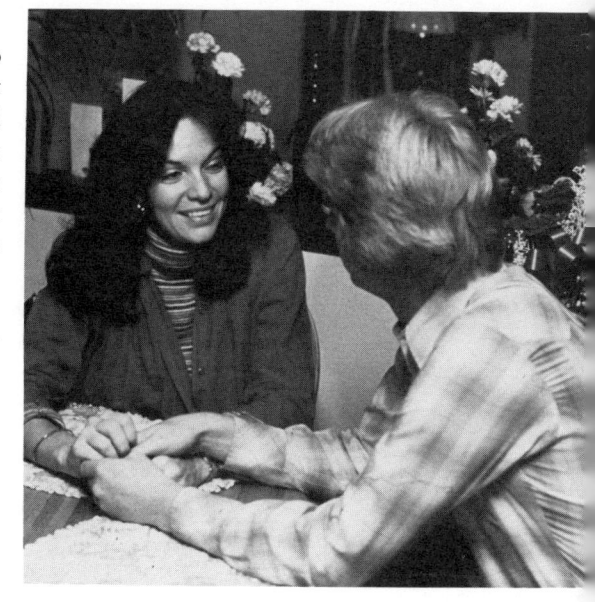

It is important for partners in a marriage to realize that no relationship will always remain serene and calm. There will always be problems and storms ahead. The health of a marriage is not threatened by problems, but by how these problems are handled. Communication skills help you become aware of the feelings and needs of your partner, to express your own feelings and needs, to define the problem that exists, to consider alternative solutions, to weigh their consequences and to choose solutions that are mutually acceptable and fill both your needs.

In our society we do not have very well-developed skills in expressing our feelings and needs. In fact, it is an essential part of our upbringing to repress our feelings and be "good boys and girls." However, until a person can express his or her feelings, they cannot change behavior. And until a person can express needs, he or she cannot ask for changed behavior in their partner. Too many times people who are married assume that because their wife or husband loves them they should "just know" what is wrong and what is needed. But it does not work that way. Problems are solved by a conscious expression of feelings and a clear definition of what one's needs are.

SEXUALITY

Effect of a New Baby on Sex

During the postpartum period you, the mother, may have concerns about your body image, resumption of intercourse, or adjustment to breast-feeding. It is common to experience changing feelings about yourself as an individual, a mate, and a mother. After birth you will need to adjust to changes in your breasts, your pelvic floor, and your waistline. Your newborn may leave you exhausted. Your interest in sex may be at a low level.

The father may well have similar concerns. You may become frustrated and overwhelmed by all these changes, and affected by your wife's fluctuating emotions.

When you bring your baby home, you may be surprised by the demands your newborn makes on your time, leaving you few moments to share together. Night feedings can leave both of you suffering from lack of sleep. You may be frustrated in your initial attempts to learn about your baby, especially in knowing what soothes and stimulates him. Exhaustion and many responsibilities may result in diminished sex drives for both of you.

A good sexual relationship is one of the most important aspects of a healthy marriage. Facing sexual difficulties caused by the mother's postpartum physical condition can lead to a new dimension of sexual pleasure if you are both open to, and understanding of, each other. Probably the greatest single reason for sexual problems during postpartum is lack of information and communication. It is important to remember that your individual needs are unique to you alone and differ from others, and that those needs will change throughout your life. Postpartum is an especially good time to get factual information concerning the physical and emotional aspects of sexuality and intercourse and to enrich your sexual life by experimenting in giving pleasure to one another with alternatives to traditional intercourse.

Sensory Pleasuring

Take time with your partner to discuss those things that excite both of you sensually. There is no one right thing—just what turns you and your partner on. Think about what attracted you before marriage. What did you find sensual about one another? What turns you on in your environment? Discuss how you both feel. Resumption of intercourse may be quite easy, or it may take a little persistence. Don't give up.

When Is It Safe to Resume Intercourse?

Physically, intercourse may be resumed when the vaginal discharge, which signals the healing of the uterus, becomes light brown and when the pelvic floor has healed enough to be comfortable. This can take from two to six weeks. Many couples resume intercourse within three to six weeks following birth; however, desire varies. Some women want to wait until they feel fully rested and confident in their mothering abilities.

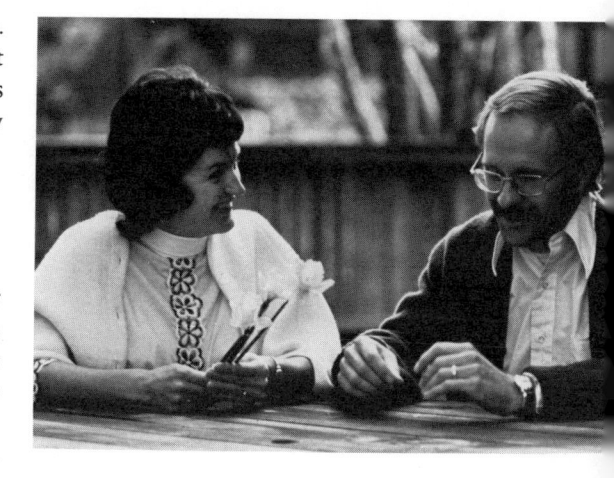

Sexuality is both physical and emotional. Even though your doctor says that you can resume sexual intercourse physically, you must take into consideration your emotional readiness.

Will It Hurt the Mother?

Both men and women are concerned about what the woman's reproductive organs have undergone during childbirth. Men have anxieties about hurting the woman when resuming intercourse. If there has been an episiotomy or any trauma to the vagina, the tissues are usually healed within a month.

It is normal for the woman to experience some discomfort in intercourse the first few times. Tension and lack of lubrication are the causes of most discomfort during the first resumption of sexual intercourse. As the woman tenses, penetration of the penis becomes more difficult and she experiences more pain. It is especially important for the couple to take special time to relax and "make love" before attempting intercourse. A glass of wine, a candlelight dinner, relaxing music, a warm bath or shower together, a massage and stroking or lubrication of the vagina and clitoris may help both of you become more emotionally ready for and excited about the experience.

Because her estrogen level drops temporarily after childbirth, the mother, and especially the breast-feeding mother, will experience a lack of lubrication in the vagina. Even when she is responding to sexual stimulation, she will secrete less lubrication than usual. Use a lubricating jelly, such as KY jelly, which is soothing, water soluble, tasteless, and odorless. You can make it part of your lovemaking; the man can apply the lubricant around the vagina, gently exploring and stimulating the clitoris. The woman can apply jelly to her husband's penis, warming it first in her hands and gently stroking it on. Lubrication usually increases when the woman's ovulation cycle begins.

Alternative Positions

Because of the trauma of birth on the vaginal tissues, especially if you had an episiotomy repair, this is the time to try different positions, to diminish pressure on the pelvic floor and deep penetration during intercourse. There is no one correct position. The position right for you is the one you feel comfortable with and the one that fits your needs.

You may find the traditional man-on-top position will not be comfortable because of pressure of the penis on the perineum. Find a position where the penis presses against the top part of the vagina and the clitoris, rather than the tender area where the episiotomy is. Some alternatives include the side-lying position, the woman on top on her hands and knees, or the woman sitting on the man's lap.

The woman-on-top position may be comfortable or it may be fatiguing for her. The man-behind-the-woman position may lessen the pressure, and allow the man to caress and stroke the woman's body. The cross position, with the man lying on his side and the woman lying at a right angle with her upper leg slung over his body and her lower leg between his legs, allows the man and woman to caress one another.

Can We Find Time to Make Love?

If your baby is fussy and his schedule unpredictable, you may find that there is never a "right time" for making love. The fatigue that accompanies caring for a newborn enervates both of you. If you are fatigued at bedtime, do not attempt intercourse. Try making love in the early morning when you arise—or even in the middle of the night after you have both gotten some rest.

When Does the Mother Begin to Enjoy Sex?

There is a difference between making love and traditional sexual intercourse. Making love is doing tender, compassionate, sensual things that turn you both on. Intercourse is the penetration of the penis in the vagina. It is important that you spend quality time in making love and let intercourse happen or not happen as a natural consequence. If you, the mother, do not enjoy intercourse or do not experience an orgasm the first few times, do not feel discouraged. This is common and okay. What is important is that you enjoy the time of making love.

Body Image

It is normal for the mother to be concerned about her body image. Her breasts may be swollen and heavy with milk, her abdomen flabby and her prepregnant weight not yet attained. It is important for her to know that she is loved—not for her perfect body but because she is who she is.

Breast-feeding and Orgasm

It is normal for a breast-feeding mother to leak milk from her breasts during intercourse. At orgasm, the hormones cause a sudden burst of milk. This may be surprising, funny, or messy.

Contraception

Early postpartum is a special period of your life. It is important to know that ovulation can take place within the first month after birth and conception is possible before menstruation is resumed. Your choice of contraceptives will be determined by the knowledge that: Birth control pills for breast-feeding mothers affect the milk supply; IUD's cannot be inserted until after your uterus is completely healed; and the diaphragm is effective only if your doctor has fitted you with a new one after birth. A double application of foam, inserted an hour or less before intercourse, is an especially effective method of contraception when used with a condom. It not only offers contraceptive protection, but also facilitates lovemaking by providing extra lubrication in the vagina.

When Will My Wife Have Time for Me Again?

It is natural for a mother to be wrapped up in her newborn. After all, its very survival depends on her and the less prepared she is for the job, the more seriously she will take the task—as she should. Again, it is important for the husband to realize that this is only a

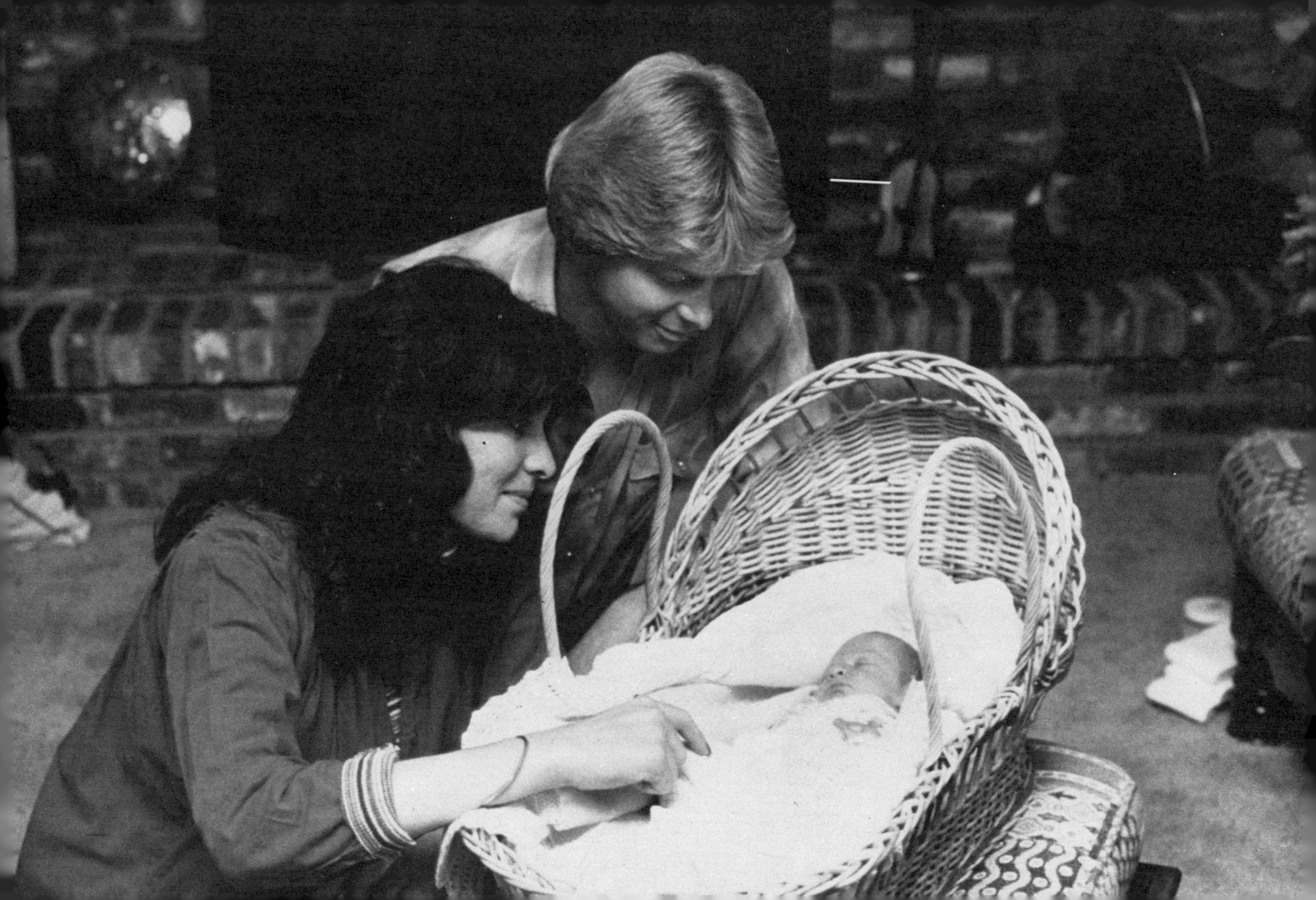

temporary period and it will pass. It is just as important that he share his feelings with the mother and not suffer them in silence.

How Long Does It Take to Return to Normal?

Couples need time after the birth of their baby to develop a pleasurable, satisfactory sex life. Your sex life will not return to exactly what it was before your baby's birth. Without compassion and communication it can be damaged permanently. With tenderness and sensitivity it can be enhanced greatly.

Not every couple can expect to work out sexual frustrations, especially during the first pregnancy. Some frustration and tension may not be resolved until after postpartum. This does not mean that your marriage is a failure. It is important to remember that postpartum is only a short period in your lives.

ENJOY BEING PARENTS

In our society parents work so hard at parenting that they forget that the most important part of the parenting experience is to enjoy yourself, your marriage, and your child. The postpartum period is soon over. After your baby adjusts to your family, and your family adjusts to your baby, you can once more take time out for yourselves. As you allow each other space to grow as individuals, your marriage is deepened and enriched.

Childbearing is a challenge, and like any other challenge, it must be met by each person in his or her own unique way. Although research gives us insights into child development and guidelines to follow, there is no one correct way to bring up a child to become a productive member of society. As you search for the best way for your family, remember that parenting is successful only if it brings you and your child health, joy, and pleasure.

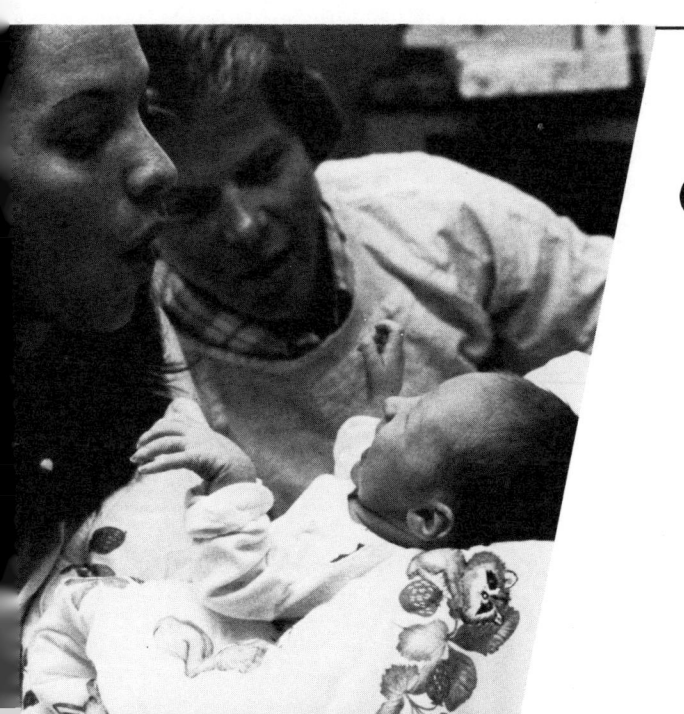

Glossary

Afterbirth: The placenta and membranes which are expelled after the birth of a baby.
Afterpains: Uterine cramping caused by contractions of a uterus following birth.
Alveoli: Clusters of glands located deep in the fatty parts of the breasts responsible for producing milk.
Anus: the external opening of the rectum.
Apgar score: A score derived from evaluating a newborn one minute and five minutes after birth. Heart rate, respiratory effort, muscle tone, reflexes and the color of the baby are all factors in the evaluation.
Areola: The area surrounding the nipple of the breast, varying in tone from pink to dark brown.
Bilirubin: A waste product composed of broken-down red blood cells which may cause a yellowish cast in the skin and eyes of a newborn (see *Jaundice*).
Birth canal: The bony passageway of the mother's pelvis and the vagina through which a baby passes during birth.
Blood pressure: Tension produced by the blood current on the walls of the blood vessels.
Calorie: Unit of heat used to measure energy-producing value in food.
Catheterization: A process which empties the bladder by the insertion of a small tube through the urethra into the bladder.
Cervix: The neck of the uterus which is the passageway from the uterus to the vagina.
Cesarean section (C-section): Birth in which the baby is delivered through a surgical incision in the abdominal wall and the uterus.
Childbearing year: The 12 months used to describe nine months of pregnancy and the first three months of the baby's life.
Circumcision: Removal by surgery of the foreskin of the penis.
Clitoris: Located above the urinary opening, the clitoris is the female organ of sexual pleasure.
Coitus: A term for sexual intercourse.
Colostrum: The first substance produced by the milk glands. A thick sticky yellow fluid high in proteins and antibodies which is the forerunner of milk.

Colic: Incessant inconsolable crying in the newborn which may be caused by gas or intestinal spasms.

Condom: A rubber sheath worn over the male penis during sexual intercourse to prevent pregnancy and venereal disease.

Contraceptive: Any of a number of methods which prohibit the sperm from reaching the egg, thus preventing pregnancy.

Cord: See *Umbilical cord.*

Engorgement: Excessive fullness of the breasts causing tenderness and soreness. Early engorgement is caused by extra fluids from blood and the lympahtic system, causing tension and blocking the milk ducts. Later engorgement may be caused by inadequate drainage of the milk ducts.

Episiotomy: An incision made at the vaginal outlet from the vagina toward the anus.

Estrogen: The hormone responsible for the growth of the uterus and of the breasts during pregnancy.

Fetal heart tones (FHT): The fetus's, or baby's, heart tones, which average about 140 beats per minute (or between 120 and 160).

Foreplay: Any form of sexual behavior preliminary to sexual intercourse.

Foreskin: A retractable fold of skin over the head of the uncircumcized penis; also termed the prepuce.

Genitalia: External sexual organs.

Hemorrhoids: Varicose veins of the anus, sometimes called piles.

Hypertension: Increased blood pressure.

Hypotension: Low blood pressure.

IUD (intrauterine device): A small plastic device inserted into the uterus to prevent pregnancy.

Involution: The return of the uterus to its nonpregnant state. This change occurs within four to six weeks after birth.

Jaundice: A yellow cast in the skin and eyes of the newborn which is caused by an excess of bilirubin in the infant's blood.

Let-down reflex: A reflex which causes the muscular cells around the milk ducts to contract and "let down" the milk into the milk ducts. This reflex is caused by the continuous sucking reflex of the nursing infant which signals a hormone to be released into the mother's body.

Lochia: The vaginal discharge a woman experiences for four to six weeks following childbirth which results from the healing of the placental site in the uterus.

Mastitis: Inflammation of the breast.

Meconium: The first bowel movement of the newborn which is black or dark green in color and somewhat sticky.

Menstrual cycle: See *Ovulation cycle.*

Milia: Tiny white spots which appear on the newborn's face usually around the nose area. They are the result of plugged oil glands and they disappear within a month.

Molding: The shaping of the baby's head during childbirth to adapt to the size and contours of the mother's pelvis and birth canal.

Neonatal period: The first four weeks of life.

Nipple: The erectile tissue in the corner of the breast which contains the outlets of the milk ducts.

Obstetrician: A physician specializing in the care of pregnant women and in the delivery of babies.

Oral contraceptive: A hormonal substance taken to prevent ovulation and pregnancy.

Orgasm: A series of muscular contractions that occur at the peak of sexual activity. In the male, these contractions are responsible for ejaculation. In the female, they promote relief of congestion in the pelvic area.

Ovary: The female reproductive gland which releases eggs and produces estrogen and progesterone.

Ovulation: The monthly release of a mature egg from the ovary.

Ovulation cycle: The monthly cyclic activity of a woman's reproductive system which consists of a building up of the uterine lining, ovulation, breaking down of the lining and, finally, discharge of the lining (menstruation). The average cycle is 28 days but can vary widely.

Ovum: The female egg cell.

Oxytocin: A hormone secreted by the pituitary gland which influences the uterus to contract.

Pediatrician: A doctor who specializes in the care and diseases of children.

Pelvic floor: A muscular sling which supports the rectum, urethra, bladder and internal reproductive organs.

Perineum: The tissue surrounding the area between the vagina and the anus.

Penis: The male organ of sexual intercourse and urination.

P.K.U. test: A test given to newborns to diagnose a hereditary metabolic disease characterized by an inability to utilize a specific amino acid.

Placenta: A spongelike organ which provides nourishment and oxygen and eliminates waste products for the fetus during pregnancy.

Postmature: A baby who is born after 42 weeks of gestation in the uterus.

Postpartum: The period of time after birth.

Premature: A term used to describe a baby born with a weight of less than five pounds, eight ounces, or a baby that is born before 40 weeks gestation.

Primigravida: See *Gravida.*

Prolactin: A hormone produced in the pituitary which is important in the production of milk.

Puerperal: The postpartum period in which involution occurs.

Rectum: The lower part of the intestine leading to the anal opening.

Rooting reflex: A reflex occurring when a baby's cheek or side of the mouth is stroked, causing the baby to turn in the direction of the stroke and root or search for the nipple.

Semen: The sperm-containing fluid which is ejaculated at male orgasm.

Sexuality: All biological, social, philosophical and psychological aspects of maleness and femaleness.

Sperm: The male's reproductive sex cell produced in the testes.

Striae (stretch marks): Stretching of the abdominal or breast skin during pregnancy causing pink or purplish streaks.

Term: The complete cycle of pregnancy at 38–42 weeks gestation.

Umbilical cord: The tube-like structure 12–20 inches in length which connects the placenta to the baby. The umbilical cord contains two arteries and one vein which carry nutrients and oxygen to the baby and eliminate waste products.

Umbilicus: The area where the umbilical cord was attached to the uterus. Commonly called the "belly button," or "navel."

Urethra: A canal extending from the bladder to the external urinary openings. In the male, it extends about nine inches; in the female the length is about one and one-half inches. In the male the urethra serves as a passageway for both urine and ejaculate.

Uterus: The female organ that receives the fertilized egg, supports and nurtures it during pregnancy and contracts during expulsion.

Vagina: The female birth canal and the organ for sexual intercourse.

Varicose veins: Swollen and distended veins in which the blood has collected and pooled.

Vernix caseosa: The white cheeselike protective substance which covers the skin of the newborn.

Vital signs: Signs which show the baby's response to life processes, including respiration, pulse and temperature.

Vulva: The external female anatomy which includes the labia majora, labia minora, and clitoris.

Womb: See *Uterus*.

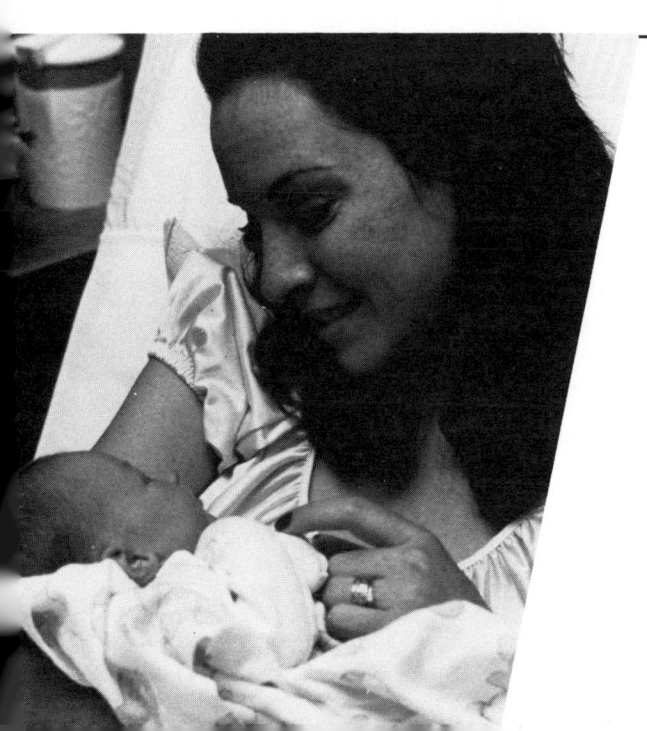

Further Reading

APGAR, VIRGINIA, and JOAN BECK. *Is My Baby All Right?* New York: Trident Press, 1973.

BANET, BARBARA, and MARY LOU ROZDILSKY. *What Now? A Handbook for New Parents.* New York: Charles Scribner's & Sons, 1975.

BARBER, VIRGINIA, and MERRILL M. SKAGGS. *The Mother Person.* New York: Schocken Books, 1977.

BING, ELISABETH, and LIBBY COLEMAN. *Making Love During Pregnancy.* New York: Bantam Books, 1977.

The Boston Women's Health Book Collective. *Our Bodies, Ourselves.* New York: Simon & Schuster, 1973.

———. *Ourselves and Our Children: A Book by and for Parents.* New York: Random House, 1978.

BRAZELTON, T. BERRY. *Infants and Mothers—Individual Differences in Development.* New York: Dell, 1972.

———. *Neonatal Behavioral Assessment Scale.* New York: J. B. Lippincott, 1973.

BRIGGS, DOROTHY. *Your Child's Self-Esteem: The Key to His Life.* New York: Doubleday, 1970.

BRODY, SYLVIA. *Patterns of Mothering: A Study of Maternal Influence During Infancy.* New York: International Universities Press, 1970.

CAPLAN, FRANK. ed. *The First Twelve Months of Life.* New York: Bantam Books, 1971.

CARSON, MARY B., ed. *The Womanly Art of Breastfeeding.* Franklin Park, Illinois: La Leche League International, 1963.

CLAUSEN, JOY. *Maternity Nursing Today.* New York: McGraw-Hill, 1976.

DODSON, FITZHUGH. *How to Parent.* New York: New American Library, 1973.

DEUTSCH, HELENE *The Psychology of Women.* New York: Grune and Stratton, 1944.

EIGER, MARVIN, and SALLY OLDS. *The Complete Book of Breastfeeding.* New York: Bantam Books, 1973.

EWY, DONNA, and RODGER EWY. *Preparation for Breastfeeding.* New York: Doubleday, 1975.

FROMME, ALLAN. *The Ability to Love.* New York: Farrar, Straus & Giroux, 1965.

FROMM, ERICH. *The Art of Loving.* New York: Harper & Row, 1974.

GORDON, IRA J. *Baby to Parent, Parent to Baby: A Guide to Loving and Learning in a Child's First Year.* New York: St. Martin's Press, 1978.

GORDON, THOMAN. *Parent Effectiveness Training: The Tested New Way to Raise Responsible Children.* New York: David McKay, 1970.

HOWELL, MARY. *Helping Ourselves: Families and the Human Network.* Boston: Beacon Press, 1975.

JELLIFFE, DERRICK B., and E. F. JELLIFFE. *Human Milk in the Modern World.* New York: Oxford University Press, 1978.

KLAUS, MARSHALL et al., *Maternal Attachment and Mothering Disorders*. Piscataway, New Jersey: Johnson and Johnson, 1974.

———, and JOHN KENNELL. *Maternal-Infant Bonding*. St. Louis, Missouri: Mosby Press, 1976.

KIPPLEY, SHEILA. *Breast-Feeding and Natural Child Spacing: The Ecology of Natural Mothering*. New York: Penguin Books, 1975.

MCBRIDE, ANGELA B. *The Growth and Development of Mothers*. New York: Harper & Row, 1973.

RAPHAEL, DANA. *The Tender Gift: Breastfeeding*. New York: Schocken Books, 1976.

REEDER, SHARON et al. *Maternity Nursing*. New York: J. B. Lippincott, 1980.

SALK, LEE. *Preparing for Parenthood*. New York: Bantam Books, 1980.

SHEEHY, GAIL. *Passages*. New York: Bantam Books, 1977.

WHITE, BURTON. *The First Three Years of Life*. Englewood Cliffs, New Jersey: Prentice-Hall, 1975.

WORTHINGTON, BONNIE S., and SUE R. WILLIAMS. *Nutrition in Pregnancy and Lactation*. St. Louis, Missouri: Mosby Press, 1977.